Contents

Preface

Much formal medical teaching and most medical texts are disease-orientated, but the practice of medicine is based upon the management of individual patients, who often do not present with clearly defined diseases. In this book we have presented a series of real case histories across the spectrum of clinical medicine 'as they happened', but structured with the aim of maximising the learning opportunities in each case.

We have arranged each history chronologically, as a series of questions and answers, which review the diagnostic and management decisions in the order in which they were made. These processes were sometimes complicated by developments in the patient's underlying condition, and this a reflection of real clinical practice. Others might, quite validly, have carried out additional or alternative investigations or varied the management at some stages in some patients, but our suggested answers are, we believe, the most generally appropriate - both in clinical practice and for examination purposes.

To use the book for self-testing purposes, we suggest that you use two pieces of thick paper or card to cover each page, and slide each card downwards to progress through each history. This 'low technology' approach can be used anywhere to allow the orderly development of the history without premature exposure to subsequent answers. For subsequent review, or for study without self-testing, the cases can simply be read from beginning to end, without the need to refer to other pages for answers to the questions. To avoid the need for repetition of 'normal ranges' and abbreviations for laboratory values throughout the book, we have included relevant normal values as a separate reference table.

We believe that the book will be of particular relevance to those working for the MRCP examination and equivalent examinations, and that it will also be a useful tool for undergraduate and postgraduate students of medicine at all stages, including those in general or family practice who are increasingly likely to become involved in the care of patients with many of these problems. The book is not, of course, comprehensive, but its 21 cases involve a surprisingly wide range of medical problems and conditions, often spanning several medical specialities.

The overall range of the book is similar to that of *a Colour Atlas and Text of Clinical Medicine* (Mosby–Wolfe 1993, Forbes & Jackson) and we hope that it will make a useful companion to that volume. Further information on most of the conditions discussed here can be found there, but this book can, of course, be used alone or with reference to other textbooks.

Acknowledgements

All the case histories in this book are based on those of real patients, although in a few cases the personal details of individuals have been modified to prevent identification. The case histories as published have been written by us, and any inadvertent errors are our responsibility alone. We were, however, greatly helped by initial drafts and illustrative material prepared by a number of colleagues and, in some cases, by their review of finished case histories. Some submitted cases had to be excluded for reasons of space, but we are very grateful to all who contributed. Unless otherwise specified, the colleagues in this list each contributed (singly or jointly) the material for one case: J Anderson, A Bridges, J Hanslip, J Gray, G Leese (2), J Mayet, F Millar, S Pringle (5), A Sands, A Seaton (2), A Struthers, D Veale (3), J Watson. We thank them all for their considerable help.

Charles Forbes
William Jackson

Normal Adult Values and Abbreviations

	SI Units	Alternatives	Approximate numerical conversion (SI to alternative)
Haematology			
Haemoglobin (Hb)	Male 13–18g/dl	mg/100ml	Same
	Female 12–16g/dl	mg/100ml	Same
Haematocrit (PCV)	Male 0.40–0.52	40–52%	× 100
	Female 0.34–0.47	34–47%	× 100
Red blood cell count (RBC)	Male 4.5–6.0 × 10^{12}/l		
	Female 3.3–5.2 × 10^{12}/l		
Mean cell volume (MCV)	80–96fl/cell		
Mean cell haemoglobin (MCH)	27–32pg/cell		
Mean cell haemoglobin concentration (MCHC)	31.5–36g/dl	31.5–36%	Same
Reticulocytes	25–85 × 10^9/l	0.2–2.0% of red cells	
Peripheral white blood cell count (WBC)	4–11 × 10^9/l	4,000–11,000/mm^3	×1000
Differential WBC			
Neutrophils	2.0–7.5 × 10^9/l	2,000–7,500/mm^3 × 1000	
Lymphocytes	1.5–4.0 × 10^9/l	1,500–4,000/mm^3 × 1000	
Monocytes	0.2–0.8 × 10^9/l	200–800/mm^3 × 1000	
Eosinophils	0.04–0.4 × 10^9/l	40–400/mm^3 × 1000	
Basophils	<0.1 × 10^9/l	<100/mm^3 × 1000	
Platelets	150–400 × 10^9/l	15,000–400,000/mm^3 × 1000	
Mean platelet volume (MPV)	7.4–10.4fl	Same	
Prothrombin time	≤14 sec (compared to normal control)		
Partial thromboplastin time (APTT)	28–30 sec (compared to normal control)		
Erythrocyte sedimentation rate (ESR)	<15mm/hr (rises with age)		
Plasma viscosity	1.50–1.72mPaS (at 25°C)		
C-reactive protein	<10mg/l	<10ng/ml	Same
Serum B12	0.09–0.44nmol/l	120–600ng/l	× 1350
Serum folate	3.6–13.7µmol/l	1.6–6.0µg/l	Divide by 2.25

	SI Units	Alternatives	Approximate numerical conversion (SI to alternative)
Serum biochemistry			
Sodium (Na)	135–147mmol/l	mEq/l	Same
Potassium (K)	3.5–5.0mmol/l	mEq/l	Same
Chloride (Cl)	95–105mmol/l	mEq/l	Same
Bicarbonate (HCO_3)	24–30mmol/l	mEq/l	Same
Calcium	2.12–2.65mmol/l	8.5–10.6mg/dl.	× 4
Magnesium	0.75–1.05mmol/l	1.51–2.1mEq/l	× 2
Phosphate	0.8–1.45mmol/l	2.48–4.5mg/dl	× 3
Urea	3.3–6.6mmol/l	19.8–39.6mg/100ml	× 6
Creatinine	44–150µmol/l	0.44–1.50mg/100ml	Divide by 100
Glucose (fasting)	3.3–5.8mmol/l	60–105mg/100ml	× 18
Bilirubin (total)	0–17 µmol/l	0–1mg %	Divide by 18
Aspartate transaminase (AST)	0–35u/l	(SGOT)	Same
Alanine transaminase (ALT)	0–35u/l	(SGPT)	Same
Creatine kinase (CK)	50–150u/l		Same
Amylase	0–180u/dl		
Gamma-glutamyl transpeptidase (γGT)	5–42u/l	(GGT)	Same
Alkaline phosphatase (alk. phos.)	20–120u/l	Several	Varies
Total protein	60–80g/l	6.0–8.0g/100ml	Divide by 10
Albumin	36–50g/l	3.6–5.0g/100ml	Divide by 10
Globulins	24–30g/l	2.4–3.0g/100ml	Divide by 10
Uric acid M	200–450µmol/l	3.5–8mg/dl	
F	150–400µmol/l	2.5–6.5mg/dl	Divide by 60
Thyroxine (T_4)	70–150nmol/l		
TSH	<6mu/l		
Cholesterol	3.5–6.5mmol/l (ideal <5.2mmol/l)	140–260mg/100ml × 40	
Osmolality (plasma)	280–300mosmol/kg		
Arterial blood gases (breathing room air)			
H^+	34–42nmol/l	pH 7.34–7.42	Same
Base excess (BE)	± 2.5mmol/l	mEq/l	Same
Standard bicarbonate (standard HCO_3)	24–28mmol/l	mEq/l	Same
Oxygen tension (pO_2)	12–14.5 kPa	90–108mmHg	× 7.5
O_2 saturation	95–100%		
Carbon dioxide tension (pCO_2)	4.5–6.0kPa	34–45mmHg	× 7.5

CASE 1:
A Female Van Driver with a Swollen Arm

A 28-year-old female van driver presented with a 5 day history of a swollen, painful left arm. The swelling had started shortly after she had lifted a heavy box while loading her van. At the time she felt no pain in her arm or shoulder and had noticed no weakness or other symptoms. She had no significant past medical history nor had she received any recent medication. In particular she was not taking the oral contraceptive pill and she was a non-smoker.

Question 1: The patient's left arm was tender. Comment on the clinical appearances shown in Fig. 1.

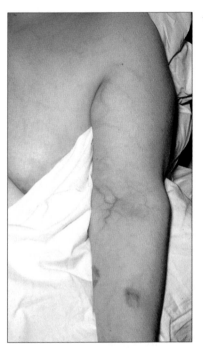

◀ **1** The patient's left arm on admission.

Answer: The left arm is swollen from the shoulder downwards (and there was a trace of pitting oedema on the dorsum of the hand). The dominant feature was a collateral venous circulation around the shoulder with the direction of the blood flow in this circulation towards the chest. There are also two small bruises on the forearm which, the patient said, were of traumatic origin.

There was local tenderness on palpation of the arm at the shoulder but movements were normal. The tender cord of the axillary vein was palpable in the axilla. There were no lymph nodes palpable in the axilla or neck. Neurological examination was unremarkable. Chest and abdominal examination were normal.

Case 1

Question 2: What is the provisional clinical diagnosis?

Answer: The provisional diagnosis is a venous thrombosis in the left axillary vein. There was no evidence to suggest any cause. No cervical rib was palpable.

Question 3: What initial investigations are required?

Answer:

Haematology

Haemoglobin	13.9g/dl
RBC	$4.82 \times 10^{12}/l$
PVC	0.409
MCV	84.8 fl
MCH	28.8 pg
MCHC	33.9g/dl
WBC	$13.4 \times 10^9/l$
Platelets	$285 \times 10^9/l$
MPV	9.6 fl

Blood film showed 'marked lymphopenia'

ESR — 140mm in 1st hour

Biochemistry

Sodium	142mmol/l	Bilirubin	5μmol/l
Potassium	4.3mmol/l	Alkaline phosphatase	101u/l
Bicarbonate	30mmol/l	Albumin	41g/l
Urea	6.3mmol/l	Protein	80g/l
Creatinine	80μmol/l	Uric acid	140μmol/l
Corrected calcium	2.26mmol/l		
Phosphate	1.28mmol/l		

Radiology

The chest X-ray and a left arm venogram are shown opposite.

Question 4: Comment on the changes in (a) the X-ray of chest (Fig. 2).
(b) the venogram (Fig. 3).

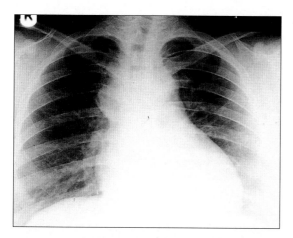

◄ **2** Chest X-ray on admission.

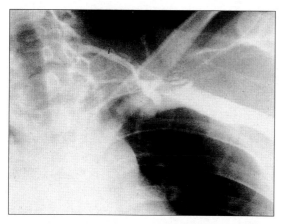

◄ **3** Left arm venogram,
2 days after admission.

Answer: (a) There is a large space-occupying lesion in the upper mediastinum, seen on chest X-ray.

(b) This upper limb venogram shows obstruction of contrast in the subclavian vein at the thoracic inlet presumably due to thrombus and there is an extensive collateral circulation. A space-occupying lesion can also be seen in the upper mediastinum.

Question 5: **What is the differential diagnosis of this upper mediastinal lesion?**

Answer: Thymoma, teratoma, bronchial carcinoma, lymphoma or retrosternal goitre.

Question 6: **What further investigations are now required to define this mediastinal mass?**

Case 1

Answer: (a) Computed tomography of thorax (**Fig. 4**).
(b) Mediastinoscopy and biopsy (**Figs 5 & 6**).

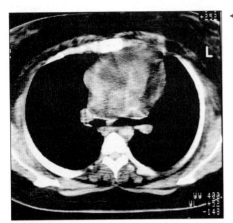

◀ **4** CT scan of thorax on admission.

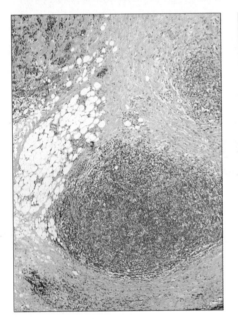

▲ **5** Histology of paraffin section of mediastinal mass.

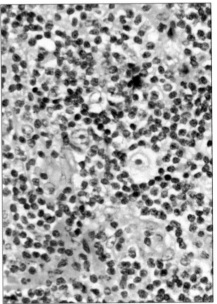

▲ **6** Close-up histology of mediastinal mass.

Question 7: Comment on these investigations.

Answer: The CT scan (**Fig. 4**) shows a large anterior mediastinal mass which is attached to the great vessels and has eroded the upper border of the manubrium sterni. There is thickening of the pericardium on the left side and this may represent tumour spread.

The possibilities are thymic tumour, lymphoma or teratoma. Mediastinoscopy confirmed the presence of a large tumour which was attached to the left lung and pericardium and had eroded the posterior surface of the manubrium. Multiple biopsies were taken.

Histology. The low power (**Fig. 5**) view of this paraffin section shows separate nodules of lymphoid tissue in fat, in areas delineated by broad bands of fibrous tissue. On high power (**Fig. 6**) the nodules are composed largely of lymphocytes but scattered eosinophils and plasma cells are also seen. As can be seen there are several large cells with clear nuclei containing prominent eosinophilic nucleoli. These are typical of mononuclear Hodgkin's cells. No classical Reed–Sternberg cells were seen. This is the picture of nodular sclerosing Hodgkin's disease.

COMMENT

The presenting feature in this lady was axillary vein thrombosis. The commonest cause of this is venous compression, usually by a cervical rib, but occasionally by the first rib, the anterior scalene or pectoralis minor muscles, or a fracture of the clavicle. Rarely, there is a congenital web in the vein. In this patient no apparent cause could be palpated. Venography showed the presence of venous thrombosis at the thoracic inlet in relationship to a large mass in the upper mediastinum. A decision was made to anticoagulate the patient with intravenous heparin while the central mass was investigated, to prevent propagation of the thrombus. Heparin is a short acting anticoagulant and can be stopped at short notice to allow mediastinoscopy and biopsies to be carried out.

Staging of Hodgkin's lymphoma traditionally follows the Ann Arbor classification (Table 1). Pathological stage is further determined by histological examination of biopsied tissues. A recommended staging procedure is shown in Table 2.

Table 1 Ann Arbor staging in Hodgkin's disease.

Stage I:	Involvement of lymph nodes in a single region (I) or infiltration of a single extralymphatic site (IE)
Stage II:	Involvement of lymph nodes in two distinct regions on the same side of the diaphragm (II) which may also include spleen (IIs), localized extralymphatic involvement (IIE) or both (IIsE)
Stage III:	Involvement of lymph node on both sides of the diaphragm (III), which may include the spleen (IIIs), localized extralymphatic involvement (IIIE) or both (IIIsE)
Stage IV:	Diffuse or disseminated involvement of extralymphatic sites (e.g. bone marrow, liver and lung)
	In addition, the suffix letters A and B are used to denote the absence (A) or presence (B) of any of the additional systemic features of fever, night sweats and loss of 10% of body weight in the previous 6 months.

Case 1

Table 2 Recommended staging procedures in Hodgkin's disease.

1.		**Required evaluation procedures**
	A	Adequate surgical biopsy
	B	Detailed history with emphasis on the presence or absence of B symptoms
	C	Complete physical examination with special attention directed to the evaluation of lymphadenopathy, liver and spleen size, and the detection of bony tenderness
	D	Laboratory studies: FBC and platelet count, liver and kidney function, serum alkaline phosphatase
	E	Chest X-ray PA and lateral
	F	Bilateral lower extremity lymphangiogram
	G	Abdominal CT scan
	H	Bone marrow aspirate and biopsy
2.		**Required evaluation procedures under certain conditions**
	A	Chest tomography of chest CT scan
	B	Bone scan
	C	Staging laparotomy including splenectomy
3.		**Useful ancillary procedures**
	A	Skeletal radiographs
	B	Gallium scan

Difficulties arise, however, when staging patients with so called 'bulky mediastinal Hodgkin's' (defined as the maximum mediastinal mass width divided by the maximum intrathoracic diameter, with a ratio of greater than one-third). Patients such as this do not fit neatly into the Ann Arbor classification, which does not take into account tumour bulk, but tumour bulk is known to be of prognostic significance. Also the criteria for extralymphatic extension (E) are poorly defined in the Ann Arbor classification; thus localized spread in the thorax, in this case involving lung, pericardium and mediastinum may be attributed to Stage IIE or IV (staging procedures showed no spread outside the thorax). The consensus at present is to allocate such patients to Stage IIE.

Stage IIE disease in conjunction with lack of constitutional symptoms suggests a good prognosis. However, anaemia, an elevated ESR, lymphopenia and relative lymphocyte depletion in the tumour mass suggests a more guarded prognosis, as in this patient. Table 3 lists the important prognostic factors in Stage I and II disease.

Treatment in this patient consisted of a combination of radiotherapy and a variant of the 'MOPP' chemotherapy regime (Table 4).

Table 3 Prognostic factors – Hodgkin's disease Stages I and II.

	Favourable	Unfavourable
Age	<40 years	>40 years
Histology	LP and NS	MC and LD
Erythrocyte sedimentation rate (ESR)	'A' and ESR <50	'A' and ESR ≥50
+ systemic symptoms	'B' and ESR <30	'B' and ESR ≥30
Clinical stage	I or II (mediastinal)	II (non-mediastinal)
Laparotomy*	Spleen negative	Spleen positive

*Prognostic significance defined by laparotomy and splenectomy.

Table 4 Principles of 'MOPP' chemotherapy.

1.	Indicated for Stages III and IV and patients with localized disease with poor prognostic features
2.	Should be given in full dose and as intensively as possible. It consists of **MUSTINE, VINCRISTINE, PROCARBAZINE** and **PREDNISOLONE**
3.	Treatment should be continued until complete clinical resolution and then for two further courses only. There is no role for maintenance chemotherapy
4.	Careful restaging is required at the end of treatment

CASE 2:
A Dilemma in Anticoagulant Therapy

A man of 67 years was seen as an emergency with a high swinging fever, suprapu-bic and bilateral loin pain and the passage of foul smelling urine which contained gas. He had obviously lost weight over several months and had a 6 month history of a change of bowel habit with fresh blood and mucus in his stool.

Question 1: What are the probable clinical diagnoses and what has caused the presenting symptoms?

Answer: This man has a fistula between the gut and the urinary tract. This was con-firmed to be a colovesical fistula by barium enema, colonoscopy and cystoscopy. As a result of the passage of faecal matter into the urinary tract, he had developed a bilateral ascending pyelonephritis and septicaemia (*E. coli* was cultured from his blood). The background disease was a colonic neoplasm which had spread locally into the bladder. Ultrasound showed a single metastasis in the right lobe of the liver. The infection was controlled by antibiotic therapy.

Laparoscopy showed extensive tumour spread within the pelvis, and local resection was not possible. A colostomy was carried out at the level of the descending colon and radiotherapy was given to the pelvis. This resulted in dramatic shrinkage of the tumour mass and improvement of the symptoms of the colovesical fistula and he was discharged home. Ten days after completing his radiotherapy the patient called his family doctor because of pain in his left thigh and calf (Fig. 1).

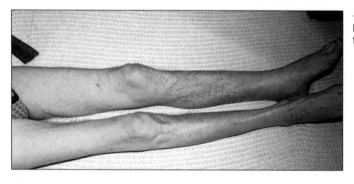

◀ **1** The patient's legs on re-admission to hospital.

Question 2: (i) What is the likely cause of this pain?
(ii) What risk factors for the likely cause of the pain are present in this man?
(iii) What investigation is required to establish the diagnosis?

Answer: (i) The likely diagnosis is deep venous thrombosis (DVT). Local pain over thrombosed deep veins is found in about 50 per cent of cases of DVT in the calf and about 70 per cent when the DVT is more proximal but it is important to remember that some cases of DVT are completely asymptomatic. As shown in **Fig. 1** the leg was swollen with an increased circumference of both the thigh and calf. There was also pitting oedema on the dorsum of the foot. There were visible superficial veins in the affected limb on the calf and thigh. The affected limb was redder than the other and it was warmer, up to the groin, than normal. Doctors should be actively discouraged from assessing for 'Homan's sign' by dorsiflexing the foot, because of the very real danger of dislodging emboli and because the test gives no additional information. Other possible symptoms and signs are shown in **Table 1**.

Table 1 Possible clinical features of DVT.

Symptoms	Signs
Swelling and tightness	Swelling with some pitting oedema on the dorsum of the foot/ankle
Tenderness to touch or movement	
Cramping pains in the calf or thigh (usually in one leg)	Pain in the calf on gentle compression in the popliteal fossa and along the line of the femoral vein
Discoloration, ranging from white to purple	Colour changes
	Increased temperature in the whole limb
	Dilation of superficial veins, particularly at the ankles
	Signs of pulmonary embolism
No symptoms in the legs: – presentation with pulmonary embolism – sudden death – detected in a screening test	No signs – the patient had been diagnosed by a screening test (usually carried out because the patient is at high risk)

The symptoms and signs of DVT are extremely variable and in about 50 per cent of patients no symptoms or signs are present; some of these patients will have no sequelae, but some present with pulmonary embolism or, much later, with post-phlebitic syndrome. As a general rule the more proximal the thrombus the more likely it is that symptoms and signs are present. The key is to be suspicious in a patient with multiple risk associations and to perform a simple screening test such as ultrasound as a routine in high risk patients.

(ii) The clinical risk factors for DVT in this man are:
   (a) Age (67 years)
   (b) Recent infection
   (c) Presence of advanced cancer, especially in the pelvis
   (d) Immobility following surgery
   (e) Radiotherapy producing tissue breakdown of tumour

Case 2

(f) In addition his plasma fibrinogen was recorded at 4.8g/l, which is extremely high and reflects the recent infection, the presence of cancer and the tissue necrosis following radiotherapy. Plasma fibrinogen is an important laboratory predictor of DVT. A range of other possible risk factors is shown in **Table 2**.

(iii) The preferred investigations for diagnosis of DVT are ultrasound and venography. The 'gold standard' test is venography, but this has the disadvantages that it is invasive, uncomfortable for the patient and time consuming. It is, however, sensitive and specific. Ultrasound is rapid, repeatable and cheaper, but it is much more operator-dependent, and therefore less sensitive and specific.

Table 2 Risk associations for DVT.

Age	DVT is unusual before 40 years of age but becomes progressively more common with advancing age
Obesity	Best measured by body mass index (BMI)
Surgery	Associated with immobility and tissue damage, for example, trauma, burns, etc. The incidence of DVT is 70 per cent following surgery for fractured neck of femur and 30–40 per cent following routine alimentary surgery
Malignancy	Often gastrointestinal or gynaecological, but most tumours have been associated. Tissue breakdown associated with radiotherapy on chemotherapy leads to additional risk
Immobility	As a result of splinting for fractures, stroke, paraplegia or any other severe medical or surgical disorder
Inflammation	Especially chest infections, inflammatory bowel disease and cholecystitis. Also after acute myocardial infarction, possibly because of tissue necrosis with an inflammatory response
Increased venous pressure/ decreased return	Results in reduced venous flow and is associated with heart failure, shock, peripheral vascular disease and pregnancy
Oestrogens	In higher dose oral contraceptive users, men receiving oestrogen (for example, prostatic carcinoma)
Haematological and biochemical abnormalities	Including polycythaemia, cryoglobulinaemia, thrombophilic states (protein C, S and antithrombin III deficiencies) and homocystinuria

Numerous clinical risk associations have been described and given 'scores' reflecting their importance, and various mathematical formulae have been produced, which can be used as predictors. The age and degree of obesity of the patient are the most important followed by the extent of the surgery to be carried out (all operations lasting over 30 minutes put the patient at special risk). The presence or absence of these factors before surgery allows for the classification of patients into high, medium and low risk and this determines the type and duration of prophylaxis to be given.

In this particular man the risks were, age (67 years), surgery, presence of disseminated cancer, radiotherapy, recent infection and immobility.

Question 3: Venography was carried out and the films are shown in Fig. 2. Describe the abnormalities seen.

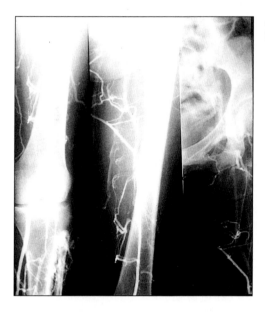

◀ **2** Venogram of the left leg at three levels: knee, thigh and inguinal region.

Answer: Contrast was injected into the veins of the dorsum of the foot and followed on the screen as it travelled into the deep vein system. This is done by applying and releasing a tourniquet at the ankle. In the first picture there are small filling defects in the network of communicating veins just below the knee. In the central X-ray the contrast has not continued in a main vein above the mid-thigh and has flowed into a collateral network of veins, suggesting an obstruction in the femoral vein in Hunter's canal. In the third view there has been some return of diluted contrast into the proximal femoral vein, which also has more proximal filling defects.

The investigation confirms the presence of small thrombi in the calf and a major occlusive thrombus in the femoral vein.

Question 4: What is the optimal treatment of established proximal vein thrombosis?

Answer: Anticoagulation should be established with a bolus of intravenous heparin (5,000 i.u.) and continued initially with an infusion of heparin at the rate of 20,000 units per 12 hours. This rate of infusion must subsequently be controlled by measurement of the activated partial thromboplastin time (APTT) to ensure that this test is prolonged by 2–2.5 times that of a control.

Question 5: What treatment, if any, should be offered for this patient's venous thrombosis?

Case 2

Answer: This patient presents a major medical, moral and ethical dilemma. With a venous thrombus of this size and position the possibility of a major or fatal pulmonary embolism is extremely high (probably 10–20 per cent). However, the colonic cancer and fistula might both be sources of haemorrhage if he were anticoagulated. An alternative to the use of anticoagulant is to insert a vena caval filter to prevent the upward migration of emboli. The deciding factor was that despite the presence of metastatic and locally invasive tumour his general health and well-being were extremely good and he apparently had the potential to have a period of good quality life with a very devoted family. The various options were discussed with the patient and his family and it was decided that anticoagulants were to be the first option, with careful control of dosage and careful observation of blood values and any blood loss. The heparin regime discussed above was started, and the patient was also started on a smaller than usual dose of warfarin (5mg stat and 5mg at 24 hours) for long term anticoagulation.

Question 6: How should the dose of warfarin be controlled and for how long should it be given?

Answer: In this patient tight control was necessary because of the possibility of colonic bleeding and this was done by measuring the International Normalized Ratio (INR) and maintaining it at a value of 2–2.5. The duration of therapy should be of the order of 3 months.

COMMENT
Deep vein thrombosis is the commonest cause of preventable death in Western medicine. In individual patients the actual cause is often not determined, but a list of risk associations is now well accepted and all patients admitted to hospital medical, surgical, and gynaecological wards should be assessed to determine whether they are at risk (Table 2).

If they are at risk and there is no contraindication then some form of prevention of DVT should be offered. This will depend on the classification of degree of risk.

No prophylactic regimens had been offered to this man for his initial laparoscopy and colostomy because of the short duration of surgery. The subsequent development of a proximal vein thrombosis was the result of a series of interacting factors.

The clinical diagnosis of DVT is difficult as the symptoms and signs are so variable. Clinical suspicion should lead to performance of an appropriate investigation so that the other pathologies which mimic DVT symptoms and signs are eliminated (Table 3).

If there are no contraindications (see Table 4) then the treatment of choice is anticoagulants. As anticoagulants have a high incidence of bleeding side effects, the importance of a positive diagnostic test cannot be overstated – i.e. a thrombus must be demonstrated before long term anticoagulant treatment is embarked on. The duration of well controlled anticoagulation should be between 3 and 6 months depending on the extent and position of the thrombus and the presence of emboli.

Table 3 The differential diagnosis of deep vein thrombosis.

Muscle strain and haematoma
Arthritis/synovitis/joint trauma
Baker's cyst
Varicose veins
Infection, with cellulitis/lymphangitis
Lymphatic obstruction, usually as a result of tumour
Swelling caused by the loss of muscle pump action in a paralysed limb
Oedema caused by heart failure, liver disease, nephrotic syndrome
Postphlebitic syndrome

These conditions may mimic the features of deep vein thrombosis. They should be excluded by appropriate investigations but it should be remembered that DVT may coexist, especially in ruptured Baker's cyst and muscle and tendon rupture. It is therefore often advisable to carry out ultrasound examination of the veins at the same time.

Table 4 Contraindications and cautions in the use of anticoagulants.

Current or recent (6/12) internal bleeding
Potential bleeding site e.g. peptic ulcer, varices, ulcerative colitis
Known bleeding disorder e.g. severe liver or renal disease
Recent stroke (6/12)
Severe uncontrolled hypertension
Haemorrhagic retinopathy (e.g. diabetic)
Endocarditis
Recent organ biopsy
Known allergy to drugs (heparin/warfarin)
Concomitant requirement for aspirin/NSAIDs

A 58-Year-Old Hypertensive Man with Dizzy Spells and Blackouts

A 58-year-old hypertensive man was referred to the medical outpatient clinic with a 4 week history of frequent dizzy spells and two blackouts. On both occasions he lost consciousness without warning and fell to the ground. He was unconscious for less than 5 seconds on each occasion and recovered immediately. There was no tongue biting or incontinence and nothing to suggest a convulsion.

His past medical history included a previous myocardial infarction 3 years ago and depression. He had a heavy alcohol intake, admitting to over 100 units per week, and he smoked 20 cigarettes per day.

His drug therapy was quinine for night cramps, sotalol and bendrofluazide for hypertension, and amitriptyline for depression.

On examination he was overweight but otherwise looked well. The pulse was basically regular but with frequent ectopic beats. Blood pressure was 188/104 mmHg. There was hypertensive retinopathy but no other abnormal physical findings.

Question 1: What is the differential diagnosis of the cause of the dizzy spells and blackouts?

Answer:

> Cardiac arrhythmia
> Transient ischaemic attack (TIA)
> Alcohol withdrawal
> Epilepsy

Question 2: What investigations should you arrange?

Answer:

> 24 hour ambulatory ECG (Holter monitoring) (**Fig. 1**)
> Echocardiogram
> Liver function tests
> EEG

His 24 hour ECG showed mainly sinus rhythm with frequent ventricular ectopics. However, while the tape was on he had a further blackout, at which time this arrhythmia was recorded.

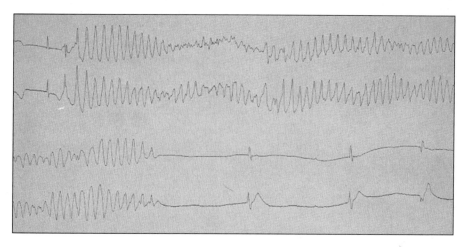

▲ **1** The patient's ECG, recorded by ambulatory monitoring during a blackout.

Question 3: What is the arrhythmia?

Answer: There is an episode of non-sustained ventricular tachycardia lasting for 15 seconds. The QRS complexes vary in height due to a continual variation in the QRS axis. This form of ventricular tachycardia is called 'torsades de pointes' (twisting of points) because of the characteristic rotation of the electrical axis of the QRS deflections during an attack.

Question 4: What are the possible causes of torsades de pointes in this gentleman's case?

Answer: Torsades de pointes usually arises when there is a long QT interval (ventricular repolarization is prolonged). Possible causes in this patient include:
(i) Electrolyte disturbance, such as potassium or magnesium depletion due to the thiazide diuretic.
(ii) Proarrhythmic effect of quinine or sotalol.
(iii) Proarrhythmic side effect of the tricyclic antidepressant.

Case 3

Question 5: What are the other causes of torsades de pointes?

Answer:

Congenital	familial long QT syndromes
Acquired	drugs – particularly class I antiarrhythmic agents, tricyclic antidepressants and phenothiazines
Metabolic	particularly conditions producing hypokalaemia, hypomagnesaemia or hypocalcaemia
Bradycardia	due to sick sinus syndrome or AV block

Other less common causes include myocardial ischaemia, CNS lesions, mitral valve prolapse, autonomic dysfunction and poisoning by organophosphate insecticides.

Question 6: What is the treatment of torsades de pointes?

Answer:

Correction of the cause
Beta blocker (without class III effect)
Atrial or ventricular pacing
Rarely, sympathectomy to remove the left sided thoracic (stellate) ganglion

COMMENT

Torsades de pointes in an interesting form of ventricular tachycardia usually, but not exclusively, associated with prolongation of the QT interval. There are two main forms of congenital or familial long QT syndromes: Jervel and Lange-Neilson syndrome, an autosomal recessive condition associated with congenital deafness and Romano-Ward syndrome, an autosomal dominant condition without hearing problems. Both are associated with an increased risk of sudden death. The underlying problem is thought to be due to an imbalance in the sympathetic nerve supply to the heart with a relative increase in activity of the left cardiac sympathetic nerves.

The commonest acquired causes of torsades de pointes in adults are drug-induced (especially antiarrhythmic agents and tricyclic antidepressants) and metabolic (especially hypokalaemia and hypomagnesaemia). The treatment is firstly to remove any identifiable causes, i.e. to discontinue the offending drug or correct the metabolic abnormality. If symptoms persist the patient should be given beta blocker therapy or, if bradycardia may be the precipitant, a permanent pacemaker. An automatic implantable cardiovertor-defibrillator may be indicated if these measures do not control the arrythmia. It is rarely necessary to consider left cardiac sympathectomy.

CASE 4:
Acute Onset of Jaundice in a Farmer's Son

This 19-year-old farmer's son was admitted as an emergency with a 7 day history of malaise, nausea, retching, and occasional vomiting. He had had episodes of sweating and shivering. The day before admission he had developed a diffuse erythematous rash over his whole body, which was most marked on his trunk (Fig. 1). On the day of admission his mother thought he had become yellow. His general practitioner was called and elicited the further history that his urine had become progressively darker and his stools were lighter than normal. He had also developed a sore throat and had some local pain on swallowing. The concern of the family doctor was that there had been a case of leptospirosis on the adjacent farm.

The key points on examination were that he looked ill, was pyrexial (38.6°C), was icteric (Fig. 2) and he had a diffuse erythematous rash. His throat was inflamed and there was mild tonsillar inflammation and enlargement. There was multiple lymph node enlargement in both sides of his neck (Fig. 3) and the nodes were discrete, tender and mobile. They were also present in both axillae and the

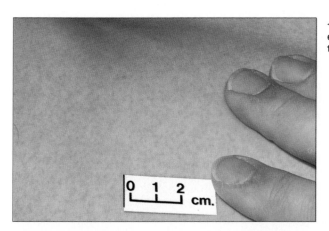

◀ 1 The diffuse erythematous rash on the trunk.

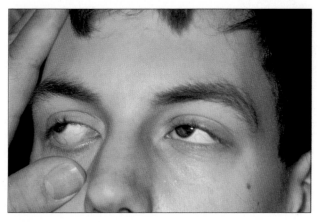

◀ 2 The patient's face and conjunctivae.

Case 4

groins, but not in the supratrochlear region. The spleen was palpable 3cm below the costal margin and was firm but not tender. The liver could not be palpated but he had some local tenderness in the right hypochondrium. Percussion suggested 3cm of hepatomegaly. There were no neurological features.

Question 1: (a) What are the possible causes of his disease?
(b) What initial investigations should be done?

Answer:

(a) 1) Infectious mononucleosis with hepatitis
2) Leptospirosis (Weil's disease)
3) Viral hepatitis

(b) a) Urinalysis   Bile ++
Urobilinogen ++++

b) Haematology
Haemoglobin 11.8g/dl   RBC 3.91 × 10^{12}/l
Haematocrit 0.35   MCV 89.5fl
MCH 30.3pg   MCHC 33.9g/dl   WBC 16.3 × 10^9/l
Neutrophils 4.4 × 10^9/l   Lymphocytes 9.0 × 10^9/l
Monocytes 2.7 × 10^9/l   Eosinophils 0   Basophils 0.2 × 10^9/l
Platelets 15.3 × 10^9/l   Mean platelet volume 9.2fl
Plasma viscosity 1.57mPaS   Prothrombin time 16sec   APTT 56sec
Blood film (**Fig. 4**)

Biochemistry
Sodium 132mmol/l   Potassium 4.3mmol/l
Bicarbonate 30mmol/l   Urea 7.5mmol/l
Creatinine 92μmol/l
Bilirubin 147μmol/l   Alkaline phosphatase 187u/l
γ-glutamyl transferase 108u/l   Glucose 4.6mmol/l
Albumin 35g/l
Corrected calcium 2.25mmol/l

X-ray of chest – Normal

ECG – Normal

Throat swab – nil on culture

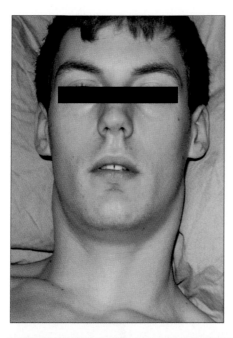

◀ **3** The patient's face and neck. Note the symmetrical lymph node enlargement (the nodes were palpable, discrete, mobile and tender).

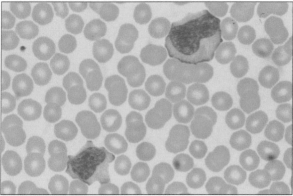

◀ **4** The patient's blood film on presentation.

Question 2: How should these results be interpreted? What is the interpretation of the blood film?

Answer: The haematology profile shows a moderate elevation of white cell count due mainly to the increase in lymphocytes, which on the blood film are seen to be activated, and in addition there is an increase in large mononuclear cells. The plasma viscosity is not increased. There is a modest anaemia which is normochromic and normocytic.

The biochemistry profile confirms the presence of hepatocellular jaundice with disturbance of liver enzymes, elevation of serum bilirubin and positive bile and urobilinogen in his urine.

Case 4

Question 3: What further laboratory investigations are urgently required?

Answer:

Serology	Hepatitis A antibody	Negative
	Hepatitis B antibody	Negative
	Hepatitis C antibody	Negative
Leptospirosis antibody		Negative
Heterophile antibodies (Paul-Bunnell test)		Positive
Epstein-Barr virus (EBV) specific antibody		Positive
Anti-i antibody		Positive

These serological tests confirm that the disease is infectious mononucleosis (IM) and that EBV is the infectious agent.

Two months before this illness this man had been seen by his doctor for a pre-employment medical examination and a routine full blood count had been done.

The results at that time were

Haemoglobin	14.4g/dl
Haematocrit	0.42
MCV	87.9fl
MCH	30.2pg
MCHC	34.3g/dl
WBC	$4.5 \times 10^9/l$
Platelets	$251 \times 10^9/l$

Question 4: What is the cause of this man's newly developed anaemia?

Answer: The cause of the anaemia is a low grade haemolysis associated with an anti-i antibody. This is reflected in the positive urobilinogen test and a subsequent measurement of the reticulocyte count (7%).

Question 5: What treatment is required for this haemolysis and what precautions should be taken when measuring haematological indices?

Answer: (a) The patient should be started on systemic steroid treatment (e.g. hydrocortisone, 200mg IV four times per day, given by this route as he was still nauseated).
(b) All haematological indices should be measured at 37°C to prevent artifacts due to red cell aggregation.

COMMENT

This case is an atypical presentation of a relatively common disease, infectious mononucleosis (IM). The typical presentation is in an adolescent with fever, sore throat, lymphadenopathy and splenomegaly, who has an increased number of atypical mononuclear cells in the peripheral blood film and a high titre of heterophile antibodies (i.e. antibodies that agglutinate sheep red cells).

IM results from infection by the Epstein-Barr virus (EBV). The virus infects B lymphocytes which have EBV receptors on the membrane (CD21), stimulates their proliferation and alters their antigenicity. This, in turn, provokes a massive proliferation of T lymphocytes, which are the majority of the atypical mononuclear cells found in the peripheral blood. These transformed T cells (CD8) are cytotoxic to the EBV-infected B cells which are destroyed.

While this is the picture of classic infectious mononucleosis due to EBV infection an identical heterophile antibody-negative disease may be induced by a variety of other infections (Table 1) and these infections are the main differential diagnosis of the clinical presentation.

Table 1 Causes of mononucleosis syndrome.

Heterophile antibody positive		Epstein-Barr virus
Heterophile antibody negative	Viruses	Cytomegalovirus
		Human immunodeficiency virus
		Influenza virus
		Hepatitis A
		Herpes simplex II
		Rubella
		Cat scratch disease
	Protozoa	Toxoplasma gondii

Case 4

The other clinical features in this young man were typical:

Fever	This is usually low grade, rarely goes above 40°C and rapidly falls to normal.
Lymph node enlargement	This is usually bilateral and symmetrical as in this case. The commonest groups of nodes to become enlarged and tender are the cervical and supraclavicular, followed by the axillary and inguinal nodes. If lymph node enlargement is asymmetrical this must give rise to diagnostic doubts.
Splenomegaly	This is to be found in about 70 per cent of cases and usually only the splenic tip is felt a few centimetres below the costal margin. It is important to remember that splenic rupture can occur and palpation should be carried out with caution.
Rash	The rash ranges from fine punctate erythema to a morbilliform pattern. Administration of ampicillin is contraindicated as it commonly results in an extreme reaction with a typical angry rash which may desquamate. Purpura may be found in about 5 per cent of cases.
Throat	In this young man there were minor changes only, but the hard and soft palates may be oedematous and there may be gross tonsillar enlargement with local oedema and the appearance of a grey exudative membrane (Fig. 5). Purpura may be found on the palate.
Jaundice	Clinical jaundice is seen only in about 5 per cent of cases and is usually extremely mild. This was the presentation in this patient. Disturbance of liver function tests is, however, extremely common, as is liver tenderness.
Neurological and cardiological	This patient had no involvement, but rarely a Guillain-Barré type syndrome may be found and even less frequently there may be ECG and biochemical evidence of myocarditis.

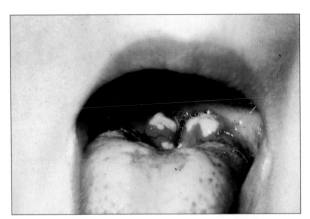

◀ **5** Severe involvement of the throat in another patient with IM. Note the presence of white tonsillar membranes, enlargement and inflammation of the tonsils and furring of the tongue.

The diagnosis of mononucleosis is suggested by the typical blood film with 'atypical mononuclear cells' which are predominantly activated CD8 T lymphocytes, but the diagnosis of 'classic infectious mononucleosis' depends on the serology. This is complex as the antibodies produced to EBV may be heterophile or autoimmune.

EBV infection produces first an IgM antibody response to the viral capsid antigen (VCA) which is evidence of recent primary infection and this is followed by IgG antibodies which persist throughout life and are to be found in about 90 per cent of the population.

The traditional test is the detection of heterophile antibodies which cause agglutination of sheep red cells, and a positive titre is one greater than 1:112. This test is, however, not specific for IM and is also positive in haematological malignancies. The test may be made more specific by selective adsorption of the test serum ('Monospot' test) and this is now widely used. Even this test gives rare false positive results in leukaemia/lymphoma.

Cryoglobulins may be found in up to 40 per cent of IM patients but haemolysis due to cold agglutinins is a rare clinical problem in infectious mononucleosis and is due to a polyclonal increase in the cryoglobulins, anti-I or anti-i, which are of IgM class. These react with red cell antigens to produce mild haemolysis. In this patient haemolysis was sufficient to significantly reduce his haemoglobin and accordingly a short course of steroid therapy was given. Such patients should be nursed in a warm room and blood samples should be analysed at 37°C. If blood transfusion is required it should be pre-warmed.

The patient rapidly responded to steroid treatment. In the clinic 2 weeks later, all the indices of infection had returned to the reference range and a rising titre of IgM specific antibody confirmed the diagnosis.

CASE 5:
Complications of the Disease or its Treatment?

A 66-year-old lady presented with pain up and down her arms and a bluish-purple colour change in her hands. Both problems were exacerbated by exercise and relieved by rest. Up until this time she had been completely well with no neurological or ophthalmic symptoms. She had complained of no trouble with her legs. She gave a history of chronic back pain, present for nearly 30 years. Her general practitioner had checked the full blood count and ESR which showed a mild anaemia (Hb=9.8g/dl) and an ESR of 90mm in the first hour. Physical examination of the hands showed both to be rather cold with a tinge of cyanosis of the nail beds. All pulses in the upper limbs were barely palpable. Both carotid artery pulses were palpable but seemed low in volume. Movement of the arms did not alter the upper limb pulses and movement of the neck produced no neurological symptoms. There were no trophic changes of the skin. The temporal artery was not palpable or tender. Neurological examination (including eye examination) was normal.

Question 1: What is the differential diagnosis?

Answer: The combination of findings is strongly suggestive of a large vessel arteritis. The likely diagnoses are:
(1) Takayasu's arteritis.
(2) Giant cell arteritis.

The patient was admitted for an arteriogram of the aortic arch, which was performed via the femoral artery using the digital subtraction technique (Fig. 1).

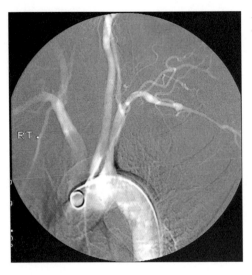

◀ **1** Arch aortogram, obtained by the digital subtraction technique.

Question 2: Describe the abnormal features in this digital subtraction angiogram.

Answer: The aorta is normal. The origins of the major arteries also appear normal, with normal diameters and walls. However, there is progressive narrowing and occlusion of both subclavian arteries with an extensive collateral circulation. Several aneurysms are seen, especially on the left subclavian artery and its collateral circulation.

The distribution of the arterial narrowing and the presence of aneurysmal dilatation favours the diagnosis of Takayasu's arteritis, although patchy involvement of the aorta is also common in this condition. Biopsy of the affected arteries was not possible without further risk to the circulation in this patient. There were no symptoms or signs in the readily biopsied temporal arteries, and no other features to suggest giant cell (temporal) arteritis. As both conditions require systemic steroid treatment, no further investigations were carried out at this stage.

The patient was started on prednisolone 60mg per day, which resulted in rapid symptomatic improvement and a reduction in the ESR to 3mm in the 1st hour. The dose of prednisolone was cut over the following weeks to 20mg per day. However, she presented acutely with fever, sore mouth (Fig. 2), and a pleuritic pain with a cough productive of green sputum. She was admitted to hospital for investigation and treatment.

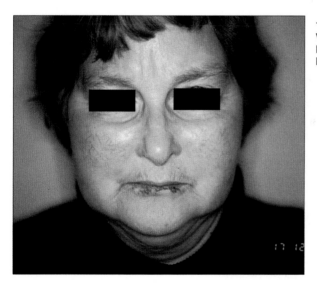

◀ **2** The patient presented with fever, sore throat, pleuritic pain and a productive cough.

Case 5

Question 3:
(1) Comment on the patient's appearance.
(2) What is the likely cause of her pleuritic pain and cough?
(3) What investigations would you carry out to confirm this diagnosis?

Answer:
(1) She has developed 'moon face', associated with iatrogenic Cushing's syndrome and she has perioral herpes simplex.
(2) Her respiratory symptoms are probably the result of pneumonia.
(3) Further investigation should include blood cultures, sputum cultures, white cell count, ESR and chest X-ray.

Pneumonia was confirmed on X-ray. She was treated with broad spectrum antibiotics and her pneumonia resolved. The dose of prednisolone was reduced to 17.5mg per day and she was started on azathioprine as a steroid sparing agent. Her ESR at this time was 42mm in the first hour. Over the next 4 weeks she continued to take azathioprine 50mg daily and the dose of the prednisolone was slowly reduced to 12.5mg per day. However, about this time, she developed severe pain in both shoulder joints associated with a decreased range of movements.

Question 4: The X-ray of the shoulder joint is shown in (Fig. 3). What abnormality is present and what is the cause?

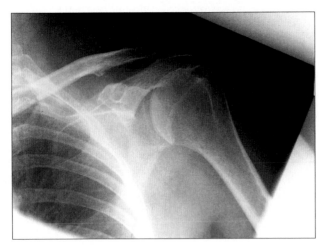

◀ **3** The left shoulder joint.

Answer: The X-ray of the shoulder joint shows a linear subcortical lucency consistent with avascular necrosis at the head of the humerus associated with steroid therapy.

The dose of prednisolone was further reduced to 12.5/10mg on alternating days. A non-steroidal anti-inflammatory drug (ibuprofen) was prescribed for the shoulder pain and gentle physiotherapy to the shoulder joints was commenced. Two weeks later she presented again complaining of pain in the lower back of sudden onset. There were no neurological symptoms or signs and tenderness was found to be maximal over T12, L1. Radiological examination was undertaken.

Question 5: Fig. 4 is the lateral view of the thoraco-lumbar spinal X-ray taken at the time. What abnormalities does it show and what is the likely cause?

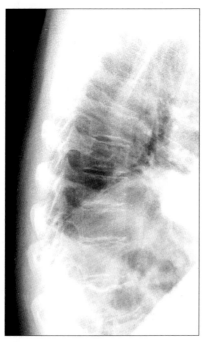

◀ **4** Lateral view of thoraco-lumbar spine.

Answer: Partial endplate collapse is present in the upper bodies of T11 and T12. There is marked demineralization of the vertebral bodies. The probable cause of this appearance is osteoporosis, which has been exacerbated by the prednisolone therapy.

The dose of prednisolone was gradually reduced to 7mg per day with no recurrence of the vascular symptoms. ESR remained low at 20mm in the first hour. The patient was reviewed in the out-patient clinic 8 weeks later and her shoulder pain and back pain had responded well to the non-steroidal anti-inflammatory drug and physiotherapy. At this time, she complained of deteriorating eyesight which was more marked in her right eye. She was referred to an ophthalmologist for an opinion.

Case 5

Question 6: What is the differential diagnosis?

Answer:
(1) Posterior lens opacity (cataract), probably steroid induced.
(2) Involvement of the ophthalmic artery in the vasculitic process. However, this is unlikely in the absence of other recurrent symptoms such as arm claudication and fatigue.
(3) An unrelated problem.

COMMENT

High dose corticosteroid therapy may be required in a number of inflammatory conditions such as systemic lupus erythematosus, Takayasu's and giant cell arteritis and for shorter periods in conditions such as asthma. In conditions requiring long term therapy it is wise to try to reduce the patient's dose to the minimum required to control symptoms and signs of the disease. Some side effects, such as fluid retention, hypertension and 'moon face' may occur rapidly especially at high doses. Avascular necrosis, most commonly seen in the head of the femur and also in the head of the humerus, is thought to be associated predominantly with high dose steroid therapy. Osteoporosis, bone collapse and cataract formation are more likely with prolonged treatment but a 66-year-old lady may already have had quite advanced osteoporosis which was further exacerbated by steroid therapy. All these complications could also have been affected by the underlying inflammatory arteritis.

CASE 6:
Tremor, Tetany and Tachycardia

A 40-year-old female unmarried primary school teacher was brought to the Emergency Department in a hysterical state with tingling in her fingers and painful intermittent spasm of her hands and feet. For several weeks before this she had been feeling generally weak, apathetic and tired but had attributed this to an increased workload and stress. On closer questioning she described perioral tingling and tingling in her fingers for several weeks, and she had also experienced intermittent abdominal pain with occasional bouts of diarrhoea. She was on no regular medication and did not smoke; but she reluctantly admitted that her alcohol consumption had gradually been increasing, so that she now drank about 1/3 bottle of vodka per day, and that she usually took temazepam each night.

Her work record had deteriorated significantly with more frequent absences for short periods, often at the start of the week.

She had complained of irregular periods 3 years ago and had been started on HRT using a combination preparation.

On examination she was crying, upset, irrational and hyperventilating. She was plethoric, had palmar erythema (Fig. 1), carpopedal spasm and multiple spider naevi (Fig. 2). There was no jaundice. She had smooth, tender hepatomegaly with the liver palpable 3cm below the costal margin, but the spleen was not palpable. Examination of the cardiovascular system showed an irregular pulse rate of 120 beats per minute, blood pressure of 120/72mmHg and normal heart sounds. The respiratory system was normal and there was no evidence of ataxia, ocular palsies or confusion.

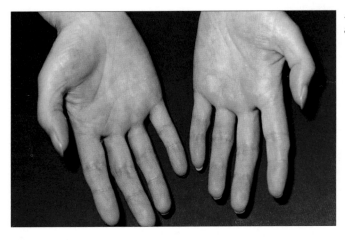

◀ 1 Obvious, bilateral palmar erythema.

Case 6

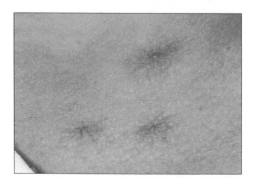

◀ **2** Multiple spider naevi – seen here on the neck.

Question 1: What is the provisional immediate clinical diagnosis and how may treatment be started?

Answer: The most likely diagnosis is hyperventilation resulting in hypocapnia and respiratory alkalosis, which causes circumoral tingling, peripheral paraesthesia and carpopedal spasm. This is best confirmed and treated by asking the patient to re-breathe from a paper bag, so that the patient inspires her own expired CO_2 (**Fig. 3**).

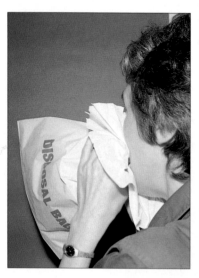

◀ **3** Re-breathing from a bag is a useful technique in the diagnosis and management of hyperventilation.

Unfortunately, although the patient settled and became less hysterical the carpopedal spasm persisted. It was clear that the patient was extremely stressed and that her alcohol intake had been increasing to at least the admitted intake of 70+ units per week. She had also developed tender hepatomegaly and some stigmata of chronic liver disease (liver palms and numerous spider naevi). It must be remembered that she was now on HRT but in view of the history and finding of hepatomegaly these signs were considered indicative of liver disease.

Question 2: What further profile of tests is required?

Answer:

Haematology	Haemoglobin	16.6g/dl		
	Haematocrit	0.482		
	MCV	102 fl		
	WBC	$6.7 \times 10^9/l$		
	Platelets	$108 \times 10^9/l$		
	Blood film: occasional macrocytes, few platelets			
Biochemistry	Sodium	144mmol/l	Albumin	38g/l
	Potassium	3.9mmol/l	Corrected calcium	1.96mmol/l
	Chloride	98mmol/l	Bilirubin	35µmol/l
	Bicarbonate	28mmol/l	Alkaline phosphatase	180u/l
	Urea	7.1mmol/l	γ-GT	346u/l
	Creatinine	106mmol/l	CK	110u/l
			ALT	320u/l
Urine	Bilirubin −ve, urobilinogen +ve			
X-ray of chest	Normal			
ECG	Shown in **Fig. 4**			

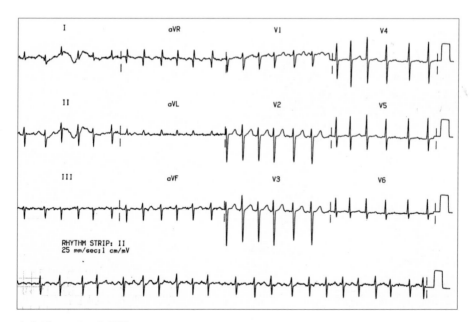

▲ **4** The patient's ECG.

Case 6

Question 3: Comment on these results.

Answer: The haematology results show a pattern typical of that seen in patients who drink alcohol to excess. The haemoglobin and haematocrit are at the upper limit of normal and the MCV is high with macrocytes being seen in the film. There is a low platelet count. These changes are probably partly dietary in origin, due to reduced intake of folate, and partly the result of a direct effect of alcohol on the red cell membrane and on the immature cells in the marrow.

Excess alcohol intake is also suggested by abnormality in the liver enzymes and by the finding of excess urobilinogen in the urine – suggesting early liver dysfunction in this lady. Of particular importance is the low level of corrected serum calcium.

The ECG (**Fig. 4**) shows atrial fibrillation, with a ventricular rate which varies from 120–140 per minute. There is borderline left axis deviation with slight anterolateral T wave flattening. The Q-T interval is at the upper range of normal.

Question 4: What additional clinical signs may be elicited in a patient who has an abnormally low calcium level?

Answer: (a) Chvostek's sign (**Fig. 5**). This involves gentle tapping of the facial nerve as it emerges from the parotid gland. In patients with hypocalcaemia this stimulus is sufficient to cause contraction of the facial muscles on that side. However Trousseau's sign is more accurate and reliable.

(b) Trousseau's sign (**Fig. 6**). This test is carried out by inflating a sphygmomanometer cuff to just above the systolic pressure for 2 minutes. In patients with a low calcium level this degree of ischaemia provokes carpal spasm.

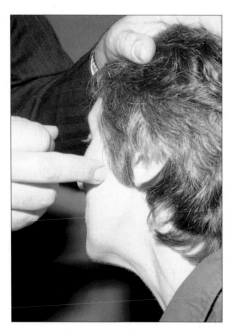

◀ **5** Chvostek's sign is elicited by tapping over the facial nerve. Contraction of the ipsilateral facial muscles is a positive result.

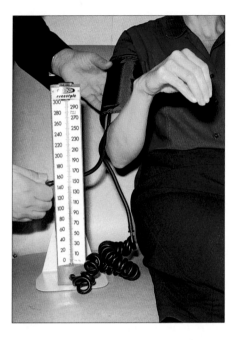

◀ **6** Trousseau's sign is carpal or pedal spasm. Carpal spasm may be provoked by temporary ischaemia of the arm. The sphygmomanometer cuff is inflated to just above systolic pressure for about 2 minutes.

Question 5: What are the most likely causes of hypocalcaemia in this patient, and how can they be investigated?

Answer: (a) Acute pancreatitis is a common complication of alcohol abuse. This lady had had severe episodes of upper abdominal pain which had lasted for up to a day and had resolved spontaneously on cessation of alcohol intake and after taking simple alkalis. The cause of hypocalcaemia in pancreatitis is probably the formation of calcium soaps in areas of fatty acid lipolysis. This is a poor prognostic sign in pancreatitis.

A CT scan of the abdomen was undertaken (**Fig. 7**) and blood was sent for amylase estimation (43u/l).

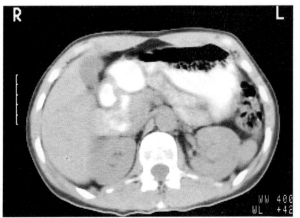

◀ **7** CT scan of abdomen.

Case 6

(b) Osteomalacia with defective mineralization of bones due to deficiency of 1,25 dihydroxy vitamin D may be associated with hypocalcaemia.
The level of 1,25 dihydroxy vitamin D was found to be 78pmol/l.
(c) Hypomagnesaemia is associated with hypocalcaemia due to impaired secretion of parathyroid hormone. Magnesium in this patient was 0.46mmol/l.

Question 6: Comment on these results.

Answer: The CT scan shows a normal pancreas and no other abnormalities. The amylase and the 1,25 dihydroxy vitamin D levels are both normal.
The serum magnesium is markedly low.

Question 7: What treatment should now be given for this?

Answer: Emergency treatment consists of magnesium sulphate infusion (e.g. 80 mmol in 1 litre 5% dextrose over 4 hours), and levels can then be maintained using oral magnesium salts such as magnesium oxide or gluconate, despite their poor absorption. The calcium level is corrected by infusing 10ml 10% calcium gluconate followed by oral supplementation with calcium citrate, lactate or gluconate.

Despite correction of the calcium and magnesium levels the patient continued to have an irregular tachycardia.

Question 8: What further management should be undertaken for this?

Answer: The patient was digitalized and the heart rate was controlled within the normal range.

An echocardiogram was undertaken and reported as follows.

ECHO   Mildly hypokinetic left ventricle with reduced fractional shortening (20%).
Mild mitral regurgitation, left atrium 4.6cm in diameter.
No thrombus seen.

Question 9: What cerebral hazard does this patient face and how should this be managed?

Answer: In this as in other non-rheumatic conditions associated with atrial fibrillation the risk of thromboembolic stroke is increased by a factor of five. The use of anticoagulants should be considered, but in this patient there was concern about:
(a) her ability to comply with instructions regarding dosage and follow-up.
(b) the altered pharmacology of warfarin in a patient with known liver disease.
(c) the low platelet count and the possibility of existing coagulation defects from failure of liver synthesis of factors II, VII, IX and X.

Anticoagulants were not prescribed and the patient was sent for DC shock cardioversion which was unsuccessful.

COMMENT

Anxiety and stress are normal components of life but this patient had excessive anxiety in association with her excessive alcohol intake. Psychological symptoms dominated her life and these included irritability, poor concentration and poor sleep and this in turn produced stress in her classroom where she had acquired a reputation for irritable outbursts. She blamed her abuse of alcohol on her anxiety and stress, but it is more likely that her anxiety and stress were the result rather than the cause of her excessive alcohol intake.

The physical symptoms from which she suffered included sweating, tremor and palpitations and a feeling of praecordial fullness. She also had some difficulty swallowing, epigastric fullness and some features suggesting the irritable bowel syndrome. These are all common features of both anxiety and alcoholism. The reason for the acute admission was hyperventilation which caused dizziness, faintness, praecordial discomfort and numbness and tingling of the hands and feet. This had culminated in carpal spasm which was present on admission and rapidly settled on rebreathing into a bag. She also complained of palpitations which probably represented episodes of atrial fibrillation or flutter.

Hypocalcaemia was found on routine biochemical screening, and in association with alcohol abuse hypomagnesaemia should also be considered. Hypomagnesaemia is often related to hypocalcaemia but the latter will never correct until the former has been treated. Hypomagnesaemia causes profound muscle weakness and can affect cardiac function. The ECG changes seen in patients with hypomagnesaemia include prolonged QT interval and a predisposition to torsades de pointes, broad flattened T waves and shortening of the ST segment.

Alcohol is often taken to help some of the symptoms of anxiety and insomnia, but it often leads to a worsening of symptoms, and these may be compounded by taking other drugs such as benzodiazepines.

The physical damage related to alcoholism can be thought of in the following ways:

(a) Direct toxic effects on tissues, e.g. cirrhosis of liver, peptic ulceration, acute pancreatitis, anaemia and fetal damage.

(b) Defective nutrition – usually of protein or vitamins causing neuropathy, cerebral degeneration, cardiomyopathy, anaemia.

(c) Infections, e.g. tuberculosis, pneumonia.

(d) Direct physical injury while under the influence of alcohol, e.g. fractures of long bones or of skull, road traffic accidents.

This lady showed many of these problems including marrow suppression, liver involvement (biopsy may be necessary for definitive diagnosis), cardiomyopathy and electrolyte disturbance.

Long term management depends on her commitment to stop drinking, which may be aided by psychosocial support. It is appropriate to involve specialized psychiatric services, which may include an initial period of inpatient care to cover the period of alcohol withdrawal. Successful long term withdrawal is dependent on patient cooperation, and is likely to be aided by appropriate counselling and/or membership of self-help organisations such as Alcoholics Anonymous. After withdrawal, this patient's medical abnormalities are likely to disappear, but continued alcohol abuse would lead to progressive liver and cardiac damage.

Dyspnoea and Chest Pain in a 59-Year-Old Woman

A 59-year-old Caucasian lady was admitted to hospital with a 24 hour history of increasing breathlessness, a non-productive cough and intermittent, sharp central and left sided chest pain which was pleuritic in type. She produced no sputum, had no haemoptysis and no palpitations. On closer questioning it was evident that she had been unwell over the past few months with episodes of dyspnoea on exertion and intermittent bilateral ankle swelling. Both these symptoms had been progressive. She had been reluctant to consult her general practitioner but had seen him just prior to admission and had been started on amoxycillin.

The only relevant history was of a symmetrical polyarthritis of the small joints of her hands (Fig. 1) and feet and rheumatoid nodules. She also had mild Raynaud's phenomenon of 10 years' duration. The polyarthritis had been diagnosed as rheumatoid arthritis by her general practitioner and had responded to the use of NSAIDs.

Question 1: What abnormality is shown in Fig. 1 and what is its cause?

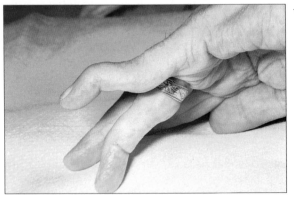

◀ **1** The patient's left hand.

Answer: The patient has swan-neck deformities of the ring and little fingers. The proximal interphalangeal joints are hyperextended, with compensatory flexion at the distal interphalangeal joints. These deformities are common in chronic rheumatoid arthritis, and result from disruption of the joints, sometimes with associated rupture of the insertion of flexor sublimis.

On further physical examination she was slightly overweight with a pulse rate of 98/min, respiratory rate 27/min and temperature 38°C. Her jugular venous pulse was raised at 7cm above the right atrium, the hepato-jugular reflux test was positive and she had bilateral pitting oedema of both legs. The liver was not palpable or enlarged to percussion and ascites was not demonstrable. Chest examination showed poor respiratory movement at the left base, which was dull to percussion and had diminished breath sounds. There were bilateral fine crepitations at both bases but these were more marked on the left side.

Question 2: At this stage what are the clinical possibilities? What emergency investigations are needed?

Answer: The differential diagnosis is:
(1) Myocardial infarction with right ventricular failure.
(2) Acute pneumonia with background right ventricular failure.
(3) Pulmonary embolism.
(4) Autoimmune pneumonitis, associated with rheumatoid arthritis.
(5) Pericarditis, associated with rheumatoid arthritis.
The following emergency investigations are necessary: arterial blood gases, ECG and chest X-ray.
The arterial blood gas measurements on air showed:

pH	7.49
pO_2	6.14 kPa
pCO_2	5.05 kPa
O_2 % sat.	85%
Bicarbonate	28.7 mmol/l

Question 3: Evaluate these abnormalities and name the overall picture.

Answer: The blood gas results show hypoxaemia, reduced oxygen saturation and mild respiratory alkalosis. This combination of findings is classified as type I respiratory failure (oxygenation failure).

An ECG was carried out in the emergency department and is shown in Fig. 2.

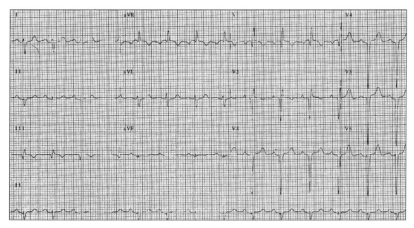

▲ 2 The patient's ECG on arrival at hospital.

Case 7

Question 4: What abnormalities are seen in this ECG?

Answer: The abnormalities include:
(1) S wave in lead 1.
(2) Inverted T wave in lead III.
(3) Prominent R wave in lead V1.
(4) Prominent S waves in leads V2–V6.

These abnormalities are indicative of right ventricular enlargement and strain.

Question 5: The PA chest X-ray in Fig. 3 was carried out in the emergency department. What does it show?

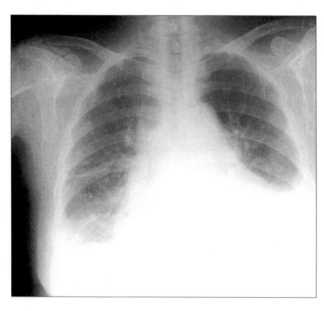

◀ **3** The patient's PA chest X-ray on arrival at hospital.

Answer: The chest X-ray shows:
(1) Cardiomegaly (CT ratio is 65%).
(2) Left pleural effusion.
(3) Prominent broncho-vascular markings at the right base.
(4) Fluid in the horizontal fissure.

Question 6: What is the next investigation of choice?

Answer: Echocardiography is the next appropriate investigation.

Question 7: What abnormalities are shown on the 2D and M-mode echocardiograms (Figs 4 & 5)?

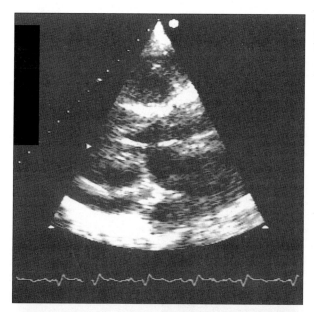

◀ **4** The 2D echocardiogram (parasternal long axis view).

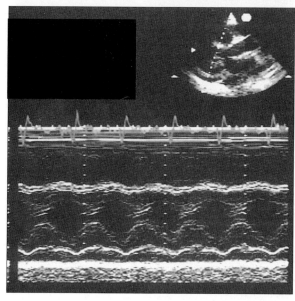

◀ **5** The M-mode echocardiogram.

Case 7

Answer: The 2D (**Fig. 6**) and M-mode (**Fig. 7**) echocardiograms show:
(1) Pericardial effusion.
(2) Dilated right ventricle.
(3) Paradoxical septal movement.
These findings are consistent with pulmonary hypertension.

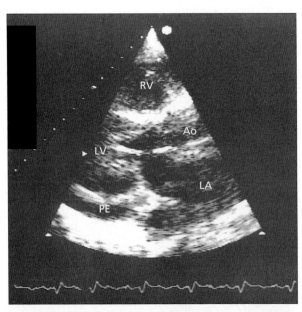

◄ **6** The 2D echocardiogram (parasternal long axis view). RV = right ventricle; LV = left ventricle; LA = left atrium; Ao = aorta; PE = pericardial effusion.

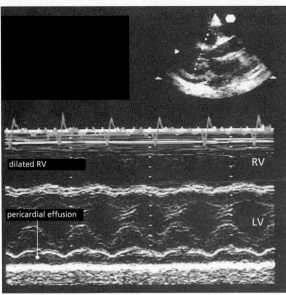

◄ **7** The M-mode echocardiogram.
RV = right ventricle; LV = left ventricle.
Note that the RV is dilated and the septal wall motion is paradoxical.

This lady was admitted to the ward and given 40% oxygen, intravenous frusemide, intravenous ceftazidime and erythromycin. Her general state improved, but she remained pyrexial and continued to have left-sided pleuritic chest pain. The white cell count was raised at $22 \times 10^9/l$ and the C reactive protein was grossly raised at 410mg/l. A ventilation/perfusion (V/Q) scan was carried out and this showed matched defects in the left mid and lower zones consistent with pleural effusion.

Question 8: What serological tests would be of value at this stage in the clarification of the diagnosis?

Answer: Rheumatoid factor, antinuclear factor, DNA binding antibody and anti-neutrophil cytoplasmic antibody (ANCA). The rheumatoid antibody latex test was strongly positive at 865 iu per ml and the antinuclear antibody was strongly positive with a speckled pattern.
These findings supported the possibility that her acute symptoms resulted from autoimmune pneumonitis.

Transbronchial lung biopsy was carried out and the histology is shown in Figs 8 & 9. The diagnosis of pneumonitis was confirmed by these findings.

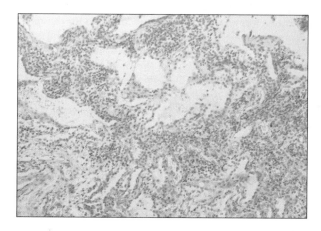

◀ **8** A section of lung stained with haematoxylin and eosin, demonstrating an extensive lymphocytic infiltrate and oedema obliterating many alveoli.

Case 7

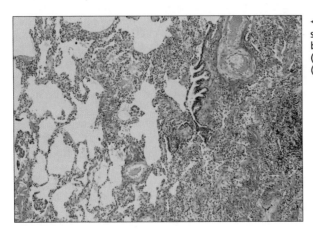

◀ **9** A section of lung stained with Marsh's scarlet blue to highlight fibrin (staining red) and collagen (staining blue).

COMMENT

This lady had a long-standing symmetrical polyarthritis and a history of Raynaud's phenomenon which strongly suggests a connective tissue disease. The differential diagnosis included rheumatoid arthritis, systemic lupus erythematosus, systemic sclerosis or an overlap syndrome with features of more than one connective tissue disease. The sudden onset of breathlessness with a non-productive cough, fever and chest pain was dramatic and characteristic of acute pneumonitis. While this may occur at the onset of the connective tissue disease, it is rare and occurs in only 3 to 10 per cent of such patients. In addition, this case demonstrated the association between pericarditis and connective tissue disease including rheumatoid arthritis. This is a more common manifestation in rheumatic disease and may occur in up to 30 per cent of patients although it is not always symptomatic. The right sided heart failure in this case was consequent on the pulmonary hypertension resulting from the inflammatory pneumonitis. This lady was treated with prednisolone and cyclophosphamide and made a rapid recovery, with a reduction in her inflammatory indicators such as plasma viscosity, C-reactive protein and white cell count, and with a resolution of her symptoms.

CASE 8:
An Unusual Case of Breathlessness

A 50-year-old female secretary was referred by her general practitioner to the local Emergency Department in an extremely distressed state. She had to sit up on the trolley because of her dyspnoea even while receiving oxygen by a face mask. She had a history of 2 weeks of gradually worsening breathlessness, progressively increasing tiredness and a 1 day history of dizziness. Ten years previously an adenocarcinoma of the breast had been diagnosed and removed surgically by 'lumpectomy', followed by chemotherapy. There was no evidence of metastatic disease at the 5 year follow up. She had remained well subsequently and had defaulted from follow-up.

On examination there was a regular tachycardia of 110/minute. The jugular venous pressure was elevated 6cm above the sternal angle, the apex beat was impalpable and the heart sounds were quiet with no murmurs heard. The blood pressure was 100/50 mmHg during expiration and 60/40 mmHg during inspiration. There was mild pitting oedema of both ankles. Examination of the breasts showed no local recurrence. The trachea was deviated to the right and the percussion note was stony-dull up to T4 level on the left side. Auscultation showed no air entry at the left base. Vocal fremitus and vocal resonance were both diminished. There was no aegophony.

Question 1: What clinical diagnosis is suggested by the signs?

Answer: The physical examination suggests that a pleural effusion is present.

Question 2: What initial investigations are required?

Answer:

Haematology

Haemoglobin	11.8g/dl		
Haematocrit	0.352		
MCV	86.3fl		
MCH	28.9pg		
MCHC	33.5g/dl		
White cell count	$17.6 \times 10^9/l$		
Platelets	$486 \times 10^9/l$		
Blood film	The red cells show anisocytosis and poikilocytisis and there are many 'tear drop' cells and normoblasts. The white cell count is increased and there are numerous immature forms. Platelets are increased.		

Biochemistry

Sodium	142mmol/l	Alkaline phosphatase	232u/l
Potassium	4.8mmol/l	ALT	42u/l
Chloride	97mmol/l	Total protein	67g/l
Bicarbonate	28mmol/l	Albumin	38g/l
Bilirubin	45μmol/l		

X-ray chest	See **Fig. 1**
ECG	Sinus tachycardia with low voltage QRS complexes due to the effusion. In some cases electrical alternans, a beat to beat change in morphology of the QRS and T wave complex, can be seen.

Case 8

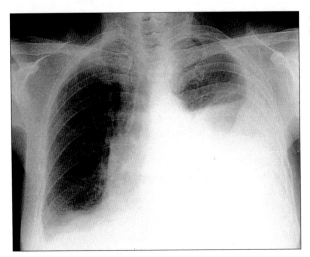

◀ **1** Chest X-ray on admission.

Question 3: Comment on these findings.

Answer: The haematology report shows the typical features of a leuko-erythroblastic anaemia, with a low haemoglobin and haematocrit, anisocytosis and poikilocytosis with tear drop red cells, high white cell and platelet counts with primitive forms in the circulation. No malignant cells were seen. In this patient the cause is probably malignant infiltration of the marrow, presumably from the previous breast cancer. The biochemical profile shows abnormal liver function with elevation of the alkaline phosphatase and a modest elevation of the bilirubin.

The X-ray of the chest confirms the presence of a very large left-sided pleural effusion which has caused some mediastinal shift. No metastases are seen in the thoracic cage or shoulders.

Question 4: What further investigations should now be done?

Answer: (a) Thoracic – aspiration of the effusion should be undertaken to relieve symptoms and obtain fluid for cytology. As shown in **Fig. 2** the aspirate was heavily blood-stained. In the post-aspiration film it was apparent that there might also be a large pericardial fluid accumulation. The echocardiogram is shown in **Fig.3.**

b) Hepatic – CT scan of the liver (**Fig.4**).

c) Bone scanning using ^{99m}Tc – pertechnetate (**Fig.5**).

Question 5: Comment on these results.

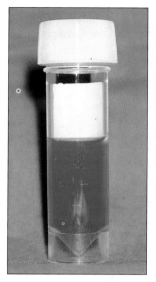

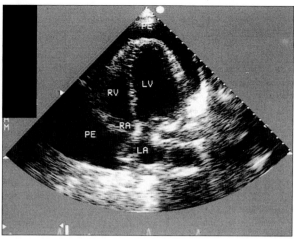

▲ **3** Echocardiogram (apical 4 chamber view).

▲ **2** Pleural aspirate.

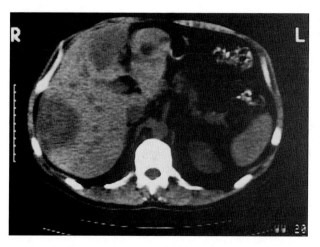

◀ **4** CT scan of abdomen, including liver.

Case 8

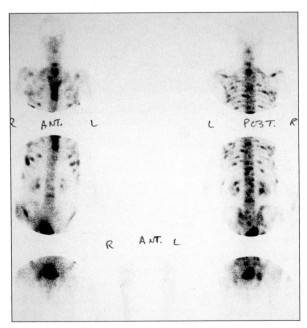

◀ **5** Bone scan using ^{99m}Tc – pertechnetate.

Answer: (a) The echocardiogram shows a pericardial effusion and also a pleural effusion – both are labelled PE; the apical PE indicates the pericardial effusion, while that to the left indicates pleural effusion. In addition there is a solid tissue mass invading the wall of the left atrium and ventricle, which probably represents secondary tumour.
(b) The CT of the liver shows multiple metastases.
(c) This radionuclide scan shows multiple bony metastases.

Question 6: What emergency treatment is indicated?

Answer: Pericardial aspiration. Cardiac tamponade requires immediate drainage to effect a reduction in intrapericardial pressure. Specimens of the aspirate were sent for cytological examination, which revealed clumps of adenocarcinoma cells presumed to have metastasized from the breast primary.

The immediate response to aspiration of the pericardial fluid was dramatic with rapid clinical improvement and normalization of the cardiac shadow size on chest X-ray. The post-aspiration ECG showed that the heart rate had slowed down and the QRS complexes had increased in size. The clinical result was a marked improvement in clinical comfort of the patient.

COMMENT
A decision was made that little could be achieved by radiotherapy or chemotherapy and management was focused on symptom control. After discussion with the family and the patient, the patient was discharged home under the supervision of the regional physician in palliative care and Macmillan (palliative care) nurses. She died without further medical distress 3 weeks later.

CASE 9:
Coma on a Winter's Night

A thin middle-aged female was brought to the casualty department at 4 am having been found unconscious in the street. The patient was unkempt but there was no smell of alcohol on her breath, no venepuncture marks, no Medic Alert bracelet and no pill bottles. On examination her breathing was slow and shallow. Her pulse was 60 beats per minute and irregular; rectal temperature was 30°C. Blood pressure was unrecordable. Neurological examination showed increased tone, sluggish tendon reflexes generally but no localizing neurological signs; the plantars were unreactive, fundoscopy normal and both pupils were fixed, unreactive to light and not dilated. Her abdomen and chest were apparently normal. There were no stigmata of chronic liver disease.

Question 1: What conditions should be thought about in this situation?

Answer: There are many potential causes of coma (**Fig. 1**), but the common causes can usually be rapidly eliminated by the history and findings on examination. In this lady hypothermia of an extreme degree is present.

Table 1 Causes of coma.

Common	Trauma
	Alcohol
	Drugs – overdose
	Epilepsy
	Stroke
	Diabetes – usually hypoglycaemia
	Subarachnoid haemorrhage
Rare	Myxoedema
	Renal failure
	Hepatic failure
	Hypothermia
	Encephalitis – viral
	Meningitis – bacterial
	Electrolyte disturbance
	Nutritional deficiency
	Neoplasia
	Hysteria
	Poisoning e.g. carbon monoxide or other chemicals

Question 2: What are the main abnormalities in her ECG (Fig. 1)?

Case 9

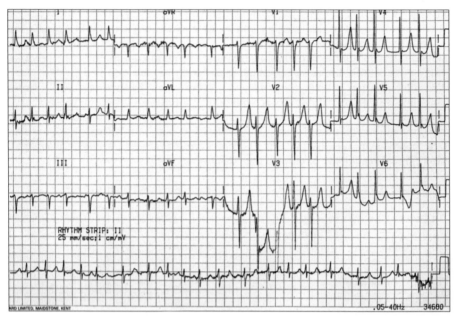

▲ **1** The patient's ECG on admission.

Answer: The heart rate is slow and the PR interval is prolonged at 0.28 seconds. In addition there are atrial ectopic beats, some anterolateral ischaemia and J waves, positive waves occurring on the down-slope of the QRS complex, and evident in most leads (also known as Osborne waves). Note also the baseline artefact due to shivering.

Question 3: What emergency management would you institute at this stage before the results of the other investigations are available?

Answer: Check that the airway is patent and administer 60% oxygen. Give IV colloid or plasma protein substitute (PPS) and change to 0.9N saline once the blood pressure has been restored. Rewarm the patient slowly (1°C per hour max) using an aluminium space blanket, nurse in a warm room and catheterize to monitor hourly urine production. Intravenous antibiotics and intravenous vitamin B complex can be considered (there have been case reports of cardiac arrest following the latter, but in this case the possible benefits probably outweigh the risks). Give prophylactic subcutaneous heparin to prevent thromboembolic complications. The patient's progress should be charted using a recognized scale, e.g. the Glasgow Coma Scale Chart.

Question 4: What emergency investigations would you organize at 4 a.m.?

Answer: Emergency investigations required are measurement of full blood count, urea, electrolytes and blood sugar, and blood gases.

The results of the tests are:

Haematology	Haemoglobin	10.5g/dl
	WCC	$16.9 \times 10^6/l$
	Platelets	$447 \times 10^9/l$
Biochemistry	Sodium	149mmol/l
	Potassium	3.8mmol/l
	Chloride	98mmol/l
	Urea	31.4mmol/l
	Creatinine	265µmol/l
	Glucose	59mmol/l
	Osmolality	360mosmol/kg
	Urine ketones	negative
Blood gases	pO_2	10.1kPa
	pCO_2	4.0kPa
	pH	7.31
	Bicarbonate	18mmol/l

Question 5: How would these results change your management?

Answer: The patient has diabetic non-ketotic hyperglycaemia as well as hypothermia. Hyperglycaemia is thought to interfere with the hypothalamic thermoregulatory mechanisms. She should now have intravenous insulin by pump (remember that the response to insulin can be altered in hypothermia). It is likely that IV potassium supplements will also be required. Serum glucose Na^+ and K^+ concentrations must all be monitored regularly.

Question 6: Which of the original clinical signs can be attributed to hypothermia?

Answer:

Coma
Hypotension
Ectopic beats
Increased muscle tone
Decreased reflexes
Unresponsive plantars
Shallow breathing
Fixed unreactive pupils

Case 9

28 hours after admission, the patient had become semi-conscious (grunting and opening her eyes to painful stimuli). She had a reasonable urine output (30ml/hour). Her temperature was 38.4°C; her muscle tone had returned to normal; there were no localizing neurological signs; her chest was clear on auscultation. The jugular venous pulse was normal and she had no sacral oedema, but she appeared to have developed a swollen, tender abdomen. A CT scan was arranged. Blood samples taken that morning to monitor progress showed the following:

Haematology	Haemoglobin	10.3g/dl
	WBC	17.9×10^6/l
	Platelets	230×10^9/l
Biochemistry	Na$^+$	155mmol/l
	K$^+$	2.7mmol/l
	Cl$^-$	114mmol/l
	Creatinine	241µmol/l
	Urea	40.1mmol/l
	Glucose	15.1mmol/l

Question 7: What is arrowed in the CT scan (Fig. 2)? What other urgent investigations are required at this stage and what changes in management would you instigate?

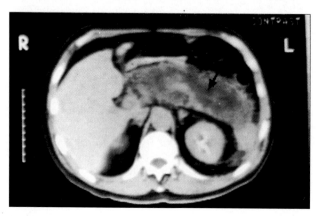

◀ **2** CT scan of the abdomen.

Answer: The arrow points to a pseudocyst in evolution in the pancreas. The entire pancreas is enlarged, and areas of autodigestion give a characteristic patchy appearance on CT. The serum amylase must be measured – it was elevated at 885 u/l, suggesting that the patient had developed pancreatitis as a consequence of hypothermia. The additional immediate management would involve inserting a nasogastric tube and aspirating the gastric contents. Her hypokalaemia must also be corrected.
Her raised temperature suggests that blood, throat and urine cultures should be taken. A chest X-ray was performed and was normal.

The patient is hyperosmolar as a result of her hyperglycaemia. The sodium concentration is over 150mmol/l, and 0.5N saline should now be given. Once the blood glucose is controlled, 5% dextrose may also be given.

During the day the patient's condition stabilized and her conscious level improved slowly. Twenty hours after admission the patient developed a temperature of 39.2°C (despite amoxycillin therapy). She had a tachycardia of 110/minute. Her abdomen was non-tender, and her chest remained clear. There were no abnormalities in her heart and she had no abnormal neurological signs.

Question 8: What would you do now?

Answer: Further urine and blood cultures should be taken, and her antibiotic therapy should be changed to cover the possibility of Gram-negative septicaemia (e.g. add gentamicin). The patient was cooled with a fan and by tepid sponging.

Haematology	Haemoglobin	8.7g/dl
	WBC	$16.5 \times 10^9/l$
	Platelets	$199 \times 10^9/l$
Biochemistry	Na+	145mmol/l
	K+	3.3mmol/l
	Cl−	108mmol/l
	Urea	19.8mmol/l
	Creatinine	161µmol/l

Question 9: What would you do on receipt of these investigations?

Answer: The haematological profile shows a significant drop in her haemoglobin and haematocrit, suggesting blood loss. The subcutaneous heparin was stopped and the patient was transfused. Subsequent endoscopy showed a duodenal ulcer with signs of recent bleeding (**Fig. 3**), and an H_2 antagonist was started. Intravenous potassium supplements were continued because of the low serum potassium.

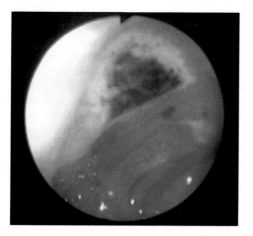

◀ **3** Endoscopic view of a large duodenal ulcer with adherent blood clot, demonstrating recent bleeding.

Case 9

The pyrexia settled quickly after gentamicin was started, and blood cultures subsequently revealed a significant growth of E. *coli*. Urine cultures were negative. The patient was established on a sliding scale of subcutaneous insulin, and given oral iron and antibiotics as well as the H$_2$ antagonist. She was then mobilized.

COMMENT

Hypothermia is defined as a fall in the body's core temperature below 35°C and it is important for accuracy that the patient's temperature is taken rectally, preferably with a thermocouple that can be left *in situ*. The normal mercury clinical thermometer is not suitable for low readings and general practitioners should also carry a low recording instrument. Hypothermia in general practice is not a common condition. It is estimated to occur about 3 times per 1000 patients in every 10 years in the average NHS practice in the UK.

Hypothermia usually occurs in the lonely elderly who are at high risk due to:

- Living alone in inadequately heated houses
- Financial anxiety over the use of available heating
- Social isolation from family, friends and neighbours
- Poor calorie intake
- Alcohol ingestion with vasodilatation and collapse or the use of sedatives or sleeping tablets
- Intercurrent illness such as stroke, Parkinson's disease, myxoedema, dementia, infections, etc.

Cases of hypothermia are also seen (especially in Scotland and Wales in the UK) by doctors who provide medical cover for Mountain Rescue Services, where hypothermia accounts for 15 per cent of all incidents in both winter and summer.

Hypothermia should be divided into mild and severe as treatment is different: mild hypothermia is defined as a core temperature between 33°C and 35°C. In this situation the patient is conscious and complains of feeling cold. There is strong involuntary shivering, peripheral vasoconstriction, tachycardia and an increased cardiac output. There may also be an increased urine output (cold diuresis) which results in dehydration.

This patient had gone beyond this stage and was in the category of severe hypothermia, which is defined as a core temperature below 33°C, and the condition had now become a life threatening emergency. Her shivering reflex had largely disappeared on admission (note its reappearance as seen on the ECG). Her muscles and joints had become rigid and muscular co-ordination was impaired. On admission she was comatose and indeed it was difficult initially to find a pulse and measure the BP. The heart rate and the respiratory rate were reduced, the heart sounds were extremely faint and the pupils responded poorly to light. In patients like this it is often difficult to confirm death. Asystole is common and the myocardium seems to be protected by the cold from ventricular fibrillation. However, attempts at resuscitation may induce ventricular fibrillation which is extremely difficult to reverse. It is very important not to diagnose death in patients with asystole until the body core temperature has risen to at least 32°C.

The prognostic indicators are the duration of cold exposure, the initial core temperature, respiratory rate, mental status, presenting cardiac rate and rhythm and the presence of any underlying pathology.

The treatment is to rewarm the patient passively or actively. Passive rewarming is performed by allowing the patient's temperature to rise slowly in a warm environment at a rate of about 1°C per hour, a rate which increases when the patient starts to shiver. Active rewarming of this patient was felt to be necessary. She was nursed in a warm room, with warmed blankets within a 'space' blanket. It is possible to speed up the process by using heat bags, airways warming or by warming the intravenous fluids. The problem with more active surface rewarming is that peripheral vasodilatation occurs and produces further core cooling which increases the possibility of ventricular fibrillation. Recently, peritoneal dialysis and cardiopulmonary bypass have been used to increase the core temperature in a controlled manner.

Initial haematological and biochemical screening tests suggested a degree of impaired renal and respiratory function in this patient with extreme elevation of the blood glucose level and osmolality. Urine ketones were negative. Hyper-ketonaemia does not develop because there is sufficient insulin secretion to suppress lipolysis and ketogenesis, but not enough to inhibit hepatic glucogenesis. The creatine-kinase and aspartate aminotransferase levels were elevated suggest-ing muscle damage from lying comatose. Such patients are often hypoxic as the low temperature drives the oxygen-dissociation curve to the left. The white cell count was elevated suggesting the possibility of infection.

The mortality in this situation is about 50 per cent and treatment must be aimed at the hyperglycaemia, hypernatraemia, hypokalaemia, hyperosmolality, uraemia and anoxia.

It became apparent in the course of this patient's illness that she had devel-oped acute pancreatitis as evidenced by the clinical signs (swollen, tender abdomen), elevation of the serum amylase and the appearances on CT scanning of the abdomen. Pancreatitis is a recognized association with hypothermia although the mechanism is not clear. In this patient there was no common aetiological factor such as alcoholism although this remains a possibility.

The pancreatitis resolved with conservative management alone.

In addition, she was found to have significant loss of blood from a duodenal ulcer, probably due to a combination of the use of low dose subcutaneous heparin and the minor coagulation abnormalities associated with pancreatitis. Blood trans-fusion was given and the problem settled with use of H_2 blockers, stopping her heparin and with the resolution of her pancreatitis.

Following a slow recovery it became clear that this patient had been abusing alcohol intermittently and occasionally heavily and was also known to buy various tablets in the pub. She required psychosocial help before discharge to the commun-ity.

CASE 10:
Acute Chest Pain in a Young Man

A 39-year-old previously fit male manual worker presented as an emergency to the local Casualty Department with a history of acute central chest pain of 20 minutes' duration. He had been at work, which involved general labouring duties, when the pain started in the region of the lower sternum and radiated into the neck, jaw and right shoulder. He described the character of the pain as 'sharp' and intermittently of a 'tearing' nature; the severity was such that he could not continue at work and an ambulance was called. There was no previous history of chest pain or recent illness.

Examination of the patient showed him to be unusually tall and thin (Fig. 1 shows him after he had recovered). On admission, he was acutely distressed and orthopnoeic. The peripheries were cyanosed and cold and clammy. He had a tachycardia of 110/minute, a respiratory rate of 30/minute and a blood pressure of 140/60mmHg in both arms. His axillary temperature was 37°C. The jugular venous pressure was elevated 3cm above the sternal angle. Chest examination showed a marked pectus excavatum deformity and on auscultation there were extensive bilateral basal crepitations found.

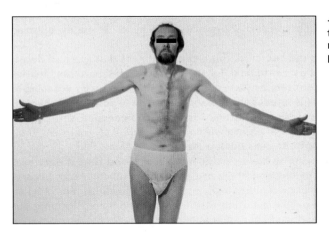

◀ 1 The patient (photographed after full recovery from the acute presenting disorder).

Question 1: What underlying clinical diagnosis is likely on the basis of the general appearance of this patient, and what other findings are possible?

Answer: The physical appearances are those of Marfan syndrome (a tall, thin male with long extremities). In this patient the arm span was greater than the height (by 6cm) and the floor to pubic measurement (i.e. the lower segment) was greater than the pubis to crown measurement (upper segment). In the hand the fingers were long and thin (arachnodactyly) (**Fig. 2**) and the joints hyperextensible. The eyes showed subluxed lenses (**Fig. 3**) but surprisingly he had never complained of visual disturbance. He also had a high arched palate.

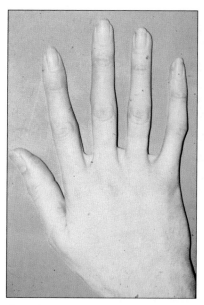

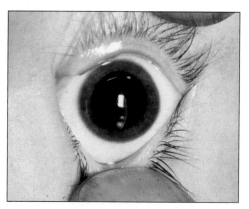

▲ **3** One of the patient's eyes. Note the sub-luxation of the lens.

▲ **2** The patient's hands. Note the long, thin fingers (arachnodactyly).

Question 2: **What was the likely cause of his chest pain?**

Answer: The likely cause of his chest pain was aortic root dissection, which occurs in 75 per cent of cases of Marfan syndrome and is the commonest cause of death. Degeneration of the aortic media produces an aortic aneurysm and dilatation of the aortic ring with incompetence of the aortic valve, which rapidly produces the features of heart failure.

Question 3: **How can the cardiovascular lesions be most readily diagnosed?**

Answer: (a) Echocardiography (either transthoracic or transoesophageal) with colour flow Doppler imaging is extremely useful for initial evaluation. The result of this patient's echocardiogram is shown in **Fig. 4.**
This is a transoesophageal echo of the ascending aorta and it shows a dilated aortic root with an obvious intimal flap (arrowed). The colour flow image shows turbulent blood flow in the true lumen (blue and orange) with no flow in the dissected lumen. This is the typical picture of aortic dissection.
(b) Computed tomography (**Fig. 5**) of the chest at the level of the aortic root confirms the diagnosis. This shows the size of the aneurysmal dilatation, the intimal flap and the false lumen (the appearances have been likened to a tennis ball).

Case 10

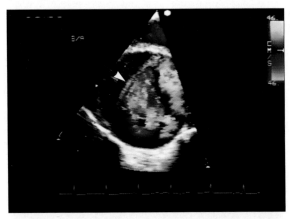

◀ **4** Transoesophageal echocardiogram (see description on page 61.

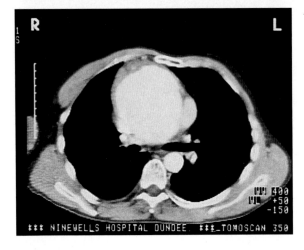

◀ **5** CT scan.

Question 4: What is the immediate management of this patient?

Answer: Intensive drug therapy should be initiated on clinical suspicion of aortic dissection alone whilst urgent steps are taken to transfer the patient to a cardiovascular surgical centre for definitive diagnosis and treatment. Left ventricular ejection velocity and systemic arterial pressure should be controlled with a carefully regulated infusion of nitroprusside. Beta-blockers were avoided in this case in view of the cardiac failure.
The patient was referred for urgent cardiovascular surgical repair of the aneurysm and valve and he made a successful post-operative recovery.

Question 5: What further investigations should be made in the family?

Answer: A full family pedigree should be obtained and the surviving family members should all be examined for the stigmata of the disease. Those patients affected should have annual examination of the aortic root for early evidence of aneurysm formation and should be treated with prophylactic beta-blockers. Prophylactic aortic surgery has also been advocated for those with early changes in aortic diameter picked up on annual screening by echocardiography.

COMMENT

Marfan syndrome is an autosomal dominant inherited connective tissue disorder with an approximate prevalence of 1 in 10,000 of the population. The variability of the clinical signs often makes the clinical diagnosis difficult. The criteria for diagnosis include involvement of at least two of the three systems classically affected (skeletal, cardiovascular, ocular) plus (usually) a family history. This patient had involvement of all three systems and a family history.

The major cause of premature death is aortic root dilatation with dissection of the aorta and the mean age of death is the mid-thirties unless the patients enter a surveillance programme. It is important in such patients to screen early in life (or subsequent to clinical diagnosis) and continue this screening for aortic enlargement yearly. They should also avoid contact sports and isometric exercises to help avoid aortic root dilatation. The regular administration of beta-blockers has been shown to retard the rate of aortic root dilatation and long term atenolol has been routinely used for this. There is evidence that beta-blockers should be started as early as 8 years of age.

When evidence of aortic root enlargement (>5cm) is obtained at the annual echocardiogram, the time interval for screening should be reduced to 3 months; and when the root diameter is 6cm prophylactic aortic root surgery is indicated, as there is now clear evidence that surgery leads to reduction of long term morbidity and mortality. The mitral valve may also be involved in Marfan syndrome, most commonly as mitral valve prolapse, and severe mitral regurgitation may occur. Antibiotic prophylaxis is indicated for dental and invasive procedures if there is evidence of valve abnormalities in these patients.

Females with Marfan syndrome are especially at risk of aortic root dilatation and aortic dissection during the course of their pregnancies due to the haemodynamic stresses this imposes. During pregnancy, echocardiograms should be performed every 8 weeks; and care should be taken to ensure that the birth is managed with minimal pushing, which raises the intra-aortic pressure.

This patient had dislocation of the lens, which is found in at least 70 per cent of cases and may significantly reduce visual acuity. Retinal detachment may also occur (in 10 per cent of patients). This patient had never complained of visual problems, and this is common as patients may never have realized what normal vision is. It is recommended that all children with Marfan syndrome are assessed by an ophthalmologist.

Scoliosis is the main skeletal complication. This should be monitored by an orthopaedic surgeon, as early surgical intervention may be beneficial.

Marfan syndrome is an autosomal dominant disorder with almost full penetrance. The defective gene in Marfan syndrome encodes a 350 kilodalton glycoprotein (fibrillin) which is an essential constituent of the elastic elements of the extracellular matrix. The gene has been identified on the long arm of chromosome 15 and the specific location is 15q15.21.9. Detection of a mutation in this gene may be used as a diagnostic aid in the 15 per cent of patients who have suggestive clinical features but no affected family members and are presumed to have arisen as new mutations. Genetic counselling should be offered to parents as they have a 50 per cent chance of transmission to each of their children.

This man came from a very large family scattered throughout Scotland. This has now been fully documented (Fig. 6) and a number of new cases of Marfan syndrome have been identified (some had already been diagnosed elsewhere).

Case 10

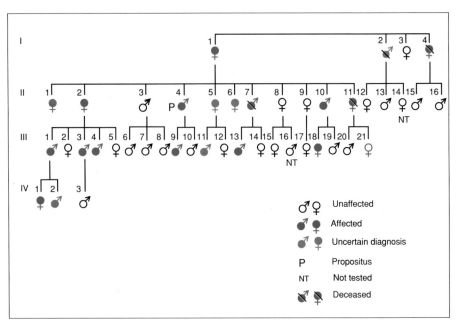

▲ **6** The family pedigree.

CASE 11:
Hoarseness and then Haemoptysis

A 70-year-old man was seen in the medical Outpatient Clinic with a 4 month history of weight loss (5kg) and poor appetite. He also complained of occasional difficulty in swallowing solid food, with a sensation of food sticking at a level of the upper oesophagus, and he gave a history of about 2 months of progressive hoarseness.

He had had a thrombotic cerebral infarction 8 months previously. At the time of his cerebral infarct he had been in rapid atrial fibrillation and he was subsequently treated with digoxin. Ultrasound of his heart did not show a thrombus, but he was anticoagulated with warfarin and his International Normalized Ratio (INR) was kept within the range of 2.5–3.5. The decision to anticoagulate this patient was taken only after careful assessment of risk/benefit, because he had two other disorders which were relative contraindications to anticoagulation. The first was long standing hypertension, but this was well controlled with captopril (fundi showed Grade II changes only). In addition he had ulcerative colitis of long standing which had been controlled with mesalazine and low dose prednisolone.

He also suffered from intermittent claudication which had become progressively more severe over the past 5 years with reduction of his walking distance to approximately 100 yards. He had been a lifelong heavy smoker but had been persuaded to give up because of his leg symptoms. He suffered from 'winter bronchitis' but his cough had not changed over this period.

Routine medical examination confirmed the presence of hoarseness but no other abnormality was found in his mouth or on head and neck examination. In particular he had no cervical lymph nodes and the trachea was central. He had features compatible with chronic obstructive pulmonary disease (COPD). He had worked in a jute mill all his life and had smoked heavily. There was a slight tinge of central cyanosis, and some evidence of peripheral vasodilatation consistent with carbon dioxide retention but he had no finger clubbing. As expected he had poor circulation in both lower limbs with cold feet, poor capillary return in his toes and reduced ankle pulses. There was evidence of slight ventricular hypertrophy with displacement of the apex beat outside the nipple line. Cardiac sounds were normal and no murmurs were present.

Question 1: What routine screening tests should be done to investigate his hoarseness?

Case 11

Answer:

(a) Haematology

Haemoglobin	15.4g/dl	WCC	$9.5 \times 10^9/l$
PCV	0.460		
MC	92.7fl	Platelets	$212 \times 10^9/l$
MCH	31pg		
MCHC	33.5g/dl	ESR	28mm in 1st hour

(b) Biochemistry

Sodium	142mmol/l	Glucose	4.7mmol/l
Potassium	4.1mmol/l	T4	86mmol/l
Chloride	102mmol/l	TSH	2.2mu/l
Urea	7.1mmol/l		
Creatinine	135µmol/l		

(c) X-ray of chest (**Fig. 1**)

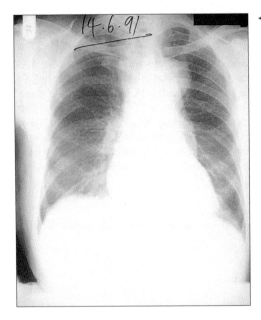

◀ **1** Chest X-ray on presentation.

Question 2: Comment on these initial investigations.

Answer: The haematological and biochemical profiles are both normal. In particular the normal levels of T4 and TSH rule out the possibility of hypothyroidism.

The X-ray of chest shows a large upper mediastinal mass which is more prominent on the left side. The lung fields are generally emphysematous and the left hilum is normal. There is some cardiomegaly (CT ratio is 55) which is consistent with his known long term hypertension.

These appearances suggest an aneurysm of the aortic arch, but bronchial carcinoma or other mediastinal tumours (lymphoma, thymoma, retro-sternal goitre and, in younger patients, germ cell tumours) are also possibilities.

Question 3: **What clinical sign should now be looked for which may help confirm the radiological diagnosis? (The astute clinician should, of course, have looked for this prior to the X-ray!)**

Answer: In aortic aneurysm the sign of 'tracheal tug' may be present. This can be demonstrated by gently holding the trachea at the level of the thyroid cartilage and extending the neck. The trachea is pulled downwards with each systole due to expansion of the aneurysm.

Question 4: **What further clinical investigations should be carried out to define the cause of the hoarseness?**

Answer: Indirect laryngoscopy showed that the left vocal cord was adducted in the midline position. This is due to damage to the left recurrent laryngeal nerve which arises from the vagus and then hooks round below the aortic arch (behind the ligamentum arteriosum) and ascends back into the neck in the groove between the trachea and oesophagus. The nerve becomes stretched and its function is defective, resulting in paralysis of the ipsilateral cord which is adducted due to the differential supply of nerve fibres to the abductors of the cord, which are more severely affected.

Bronchoscopy was also carried out at this time and showed evidence of a pulsatile mass compressing the left main stem bronchus.

Question 5: **What imaging technique should now be done to more accurately define the lesion?**

Answer: Computed tomography (unenhanced and enhanced) is required. **Figs 2 & 3** show cuts made at the level of the aortic arch (unenhanced and enhanced). **Fig. 4** is an enhanced slice to show the heart and descending aorta.

Case 11

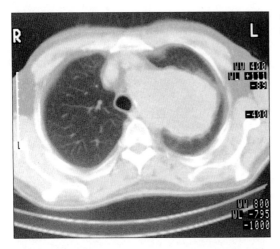

◀ **2** Unenhanced CT scan at level of aortic arch.

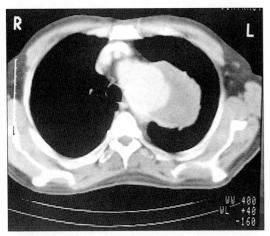

◀ **3** Enhanced CT scan at level of aortic arch.

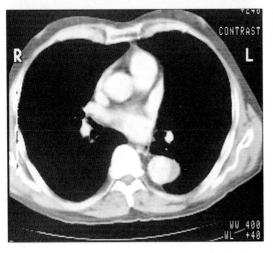

◀ **4** Enhanced CT scan, including descending aorta.

Question 6: What does CT scanning show?

Answer: CT scanning shows an extensive aneurysm of the aortic arch which is full of thrombus which does not enhance. The enhanced part of the descending aorta is not concentric with and within the unenhanced wall. This represents a dissection of the descending thoracic aorta.

As a result of the findings a decision was made to stop his warfarin therapy but before this could be done he developed a major haemoptysis, producing about 400ml of fresh bright red blood. His haemoglobin was now 9g/dl, suggesting that subclinical bleeding had preceded this acute event. The patient was admitted, cross matched and blood transfusion initiated. A decision was made to reverse his anticoagulants.

Question 7: What is the emergency method of reversal of warfarin action?

Answer: Ten milligrams of a water soluble preparation of vitamin K_1 is given intra-venously, but this is a relatively slow method of reversal of warfarin action. In the presence of active bleeding an infusion of a heat treated concentrate of vitamin-K dependent factors should also be given. This instantly corrected the coagulation defect in this patient and the vitamin K_1 antagonized the longer-term action of warfarin.

As part of his assessment for surgery a further X-ray of the chest was undertaken.

Question 8: What does the X-ray (Fig. 5) show? Compare it with Fig. 1, which was taken 5 weeks previously.

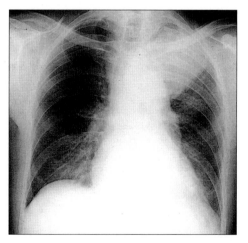

◀ **5** Chest X-ray 5 weeks after first pre-sentation.

Case 11

Answer: There has been a very significant increase in size of the lesion in the left upper zone. This was felt to be due to enlargement of the aneurysm in association with consolidation of the apex of the left lung.

Because of the life threatening situation a decision was made for him to have emergency surgery.

Question 9: **What additional imaging is required to define the potential scope of surgery?**

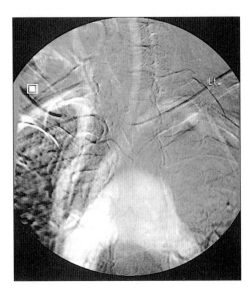

◀ **6** Digital subtraction angiogram, demonstrating the extent of the aneurysm.

Answer: Digital subtraction angiography (**Fig. 6**). This demonstrates the extent of the aneurysm, which arises distal to the origin of the left subclavian artery; this is of major practical importance as surgery is feasible without the need for cardiac bypass.

At operation a circular defect was found in the aneurysmal wall which was sealed by adhesion to the upper lobe of the left lung into which it had eroded. The adjacent lung substance was full of thrombus and this explained the radiological appearances.

Fig. 7 is a per-operative photograph. The aorta has been incised and the surgeon's finger is retracting the vessel wall. The irregular structure seen inside is lung parenchyma which had sealed the defect in the aortic wall. The aneurysmal defect was replaced by a Dacron graft. Post operatively the patient was noted to have faecal and urinary incontinence and a flaccid paraparesis.

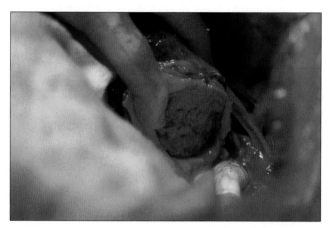

◀ 7 Per-operative photograph.

Question 10: What has caused the postoperative complications and what is the prognosis?

Answer: Damage to spinal arteries during grafting and also during the clamping period has produced ischaemia of the cord. This is a recognized complication of the procedure but often these symptoms and signs resolve completely.

COMMENT

Historically, syphilitic infection was the usual cause of aneurysms of the thoracic aorta, usually in the ascending aorta. This is now very rare; the commonest cause is atheromatous degeneration, and the aneurysm may be in the ascending aorta, the arch or the descending aorta. This patient was known to have had peripheral vascular disease and a previous stroke so it was likely that the aetiology was atheromatous. The syphilitic serology profile was negative and there were no other clinical stigmata of this infection. Histology of the surgical specimen confirmed the underlying cause.

The clinical presentation was with damage to the left recurrent laryngeal nerve and some oesophageal compression. Bronchoscopy revealed the involvement of the left main stem bronchus but he did not have the typical 'brassy' cough or stridor at that time and he never had the anterior chest pain which might have been expected in someone with such advanced disease.

Case 11

Erosion of adjacent structures is inevitable and the presentation may result from rupture into the oesophagus, trachea or lung due to erosion of the normal tissue by the expanding aneurysm. In this case haemoptysis resulted from erosion into the left lung, the compressed tissue of which limited the degree of blood loss when rupture eventually occurred.

A variety of imaging modalities may be used to confirm the clinical suspicion of aneurysm. These include CT, angiography, cardiac ultrasound and MRI, which are all of value in showing the size of the lesion, the presence of thrombus in the aneurysmal sac, the compression of surrounding structures and involvement of related branching blood vessels. This definition allows the surgeon to plan the extent of his surgery accurately.

In this patient there was also evidence of aortic dissection, which may have been in part due to his taking oral anticoagulants as well as to the degeneration of the aortic wall structures.

Treatment of an aneurysm of this size is always surgical after stabilization of all the relevant medical problems.

CASE 12:
Back Pain in an Elderly Woman

A 79-year-old previously fit female patient presented with a 2 month history of mid-thoracic back pain which felt 'like a tight corset' and was severe enough to interrupt her sleep. In addition, she was nauseated, her appetite was impaired and she had lost 3kg in weight. In the 24 hours prior to admission she had trouble standing, walking and getting out of her chair and this had resulted in two falls. She was aware of a numb sensation in both her legs. There was no sphincter disturbance. Her only medications at this time were analgesics for her back pain and night sedation. She had no past medical history of note, was a non-smoker and teetotal.

On examination there was tenderness over her mid-thoracic spine. The power in her limbs was normal, apart from weak dorsiflexion at her right ankle. The tone was increased in both lower limbs, with brisk ankle and knee reflexes and bilateral extensor plantar responses. Light touch sensation was normal, but pin prick sensation revealed a sensory level at T6. Vibration sense was absent in the lower limbs, proprioception was impaired, and co-ordination was poor.

Question 1: What are the possible causes of her neurological deficit?

Answer: The features are suggestive of spinal cord compression at the level of T6 and this is likely to be associated with collapse of the vertebral body or protrusion of a disc. The history of weight loss may suggest tumour as a likely cause although TB is also a possibility. Clinically there was no obvious site of a primary lesion.

Question 2: What initial investigations are called for?

Answer:

Haematology		
Haemoglobin	11.7g/dl	
WBC	5.5×10^9/l	
Platelets	249×10^9/l	
ESR	68mm in 1st hour	
Blood film	Marked rouleaux formation	
	Normochromic, normocytic cells	
Biochemistry		
Sodium	136mmol/l	
Potassium	4.0mmol/l	
Urea	5.3mmol/l	
Creatinine	104µmol/l	
Total protein	68g/l	
Albumin	33g/l	
Corrected calcium	2.36mmol/l	
Alkaline phosphatase	127 units/l	
Urate	360 µmol/l	
Radiology		
Chest X-ray	Normal	
Dorsal spine X-ray	**Fig. 1**	

Case 12

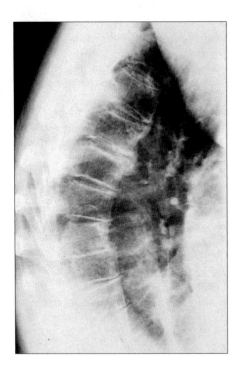

Question 3: What abnormalities are present in the lateral view of the spine (Fig. 1)?

Answer: The spine shows evidence of osteoarthritis of long standing, the vertebral bodies are generally osteoporotic, there is early anterior wedging of the T6 body which appears sclerotic and there is erosion of the pedicles. There are osteolytic areas in the other vertebral bodies.

Question 4: What are the most likely diagnoses?

Answer: Sclerosis and erosion of T6 could result from secondary deposits from an unknown primary tumour, but the presence of multiple lytic lesions in other vertebrae suggests the possibility of multiple myeloma. This possibility is strengthened by the finding of moderate anaemia, an elevated ESR and rouleaux formation on the blood film.

Question 5: What further investigations would you perform?

Answer:
Radiology
    Skeletal survey to include skull, pelvis, and long bones
    CT scan of the spinal segment affected
    CT scan of abdomen
    Serum and urine electrophoresis
    Bone marrow examination

Question 6: Comment on the appearances of
(a) The skull (Fig. 2)
(b) Transverse CT of T6 vertebra (Fig. 3)
(c) CT of abdomen (Fig. 4)

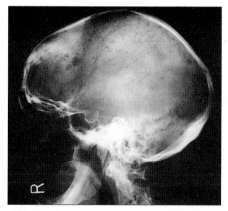

▲ **2** Lateral view of the skull.

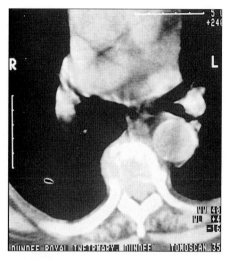

▲ **3** Transverse CT scan at level of T6 vertebra.

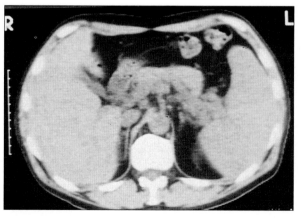

◀ **4** CT scan of abdomen at level of liver and spleen.

Case 12

Answer: (a) The lateral view of the skull shows typical punched out lesions without surrounding sclerosis. This is characteristic of multiple myeloma deposits and is rarely seen with other secondary tumours.

(b) The CT scan of the T6 vertebra shows generalized loss of normal bone with extensive bone lysis and extension of the tumour process into the spinal canal.

(c) The abdominal CT scan shows splenomegaly which was not found on clinical examination.

Question 7: Comment on the serum electrophoresis (Fig. 5).

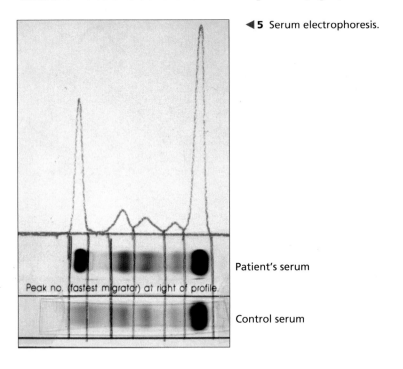

◀5 Serum electrophoresis.

Patient's serum

Peak no. (fastest migrator) at right of profile.

Control serum

Answer: Electrophoresis of the serum was carried out to confirm the presence of an M band. This is clearly seen to the left in the patient's serum (above). Further analysis of this showed it to be an IgG paraprotein, present at a concentration of 17g/l. Bence Jones proteinuria was also present, as was confirmed by heating the urine and by electrophoresis of concentrated urine.

Question 8: What diagnostic features are seen in the marrow smears (Figs 6 & 7)?

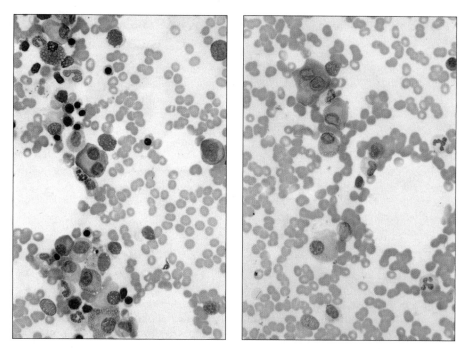

▲ **6 & 7** Bone marrow films. These views are taken from the edge of the marrow smear to show individual cells.

Answer: The bone marrow is generally hypercellular and contains an excess of diverse plasma cells (myeloma cells). Some of the myeloma cells are large, with immature-looking chromatin, while some are smaller, with clumping of the chromatin. The cytoplasm is often pale. Multinucleate cells are also present. There are Russell bodies in the cytoplasm, representing accumulations of IgG.

Question 9: What features of multiple myeloma are associated with a poor prognosis?

Answer:
- Advancing years.
- Severe anaemia.
- Low serum albumin.
- Renal impairment.
- High serum calcium.
- High levels of lambda light chains.
- Extensive osteolytic lesions/total myeloma cell mass.
- High monoclonal component.
- High β_2-microglobulin levels.
- Expression of CD10 antigen on the cells.
- Active mitosis of plasma cells.

Case 12

Question 10: What are the broad principles of patient management in myeloma?

Answer:
• Maintain mobility and a high fluid intake to prevent hypercalcaemia, renal failure and hyperviscosity-related problems.
• Control pain with adequate analgesia.
• Relieve lesions with local effects (such as cord compression in this patient) by radiotherapy.
• The usual specific therapy for multiple myeloma is melphalan (an alkylating agent) in a dose of 7mg/m^2/day for 4 days every 3 weeks.
• Therapy should be monitored with special attention to the haematological profile (especially haemoglobin and white cells) and biochemistry (especially renal function, calcium and levels of the M-protein). Successful therapy is also indicated by a falling β_2-microglobulin and disappearance of light chain proteinuria.
• If hypercalcaemia occurs, treatment with steroids or other calcium-lowering agents may be required.

COMMENT
Multiple myeloma is the result of malignant B cell proliferation, which usually occurs in the marrow with the production of mainly plasma cells, which produce excessive amounts of paraproteins. It almost always presents in the middle-aged or elderly, and is rarely seen below the age of 40 years. According to Hodgkin the average general practice in the UK will see 2 cases in 10 years for every 1000 patients on its list. Clinical presentations result from (a) the uncontrolled proliferation of plasma cells with subsequent effects on the marrow and the skeleton (b) the subsequent plasma protein abnormalities, mainly paraproteins, causing hyperviscosity syndromes (presenting as a bleeding tendency or as tissue ischaemia) or hypogamma-globulinaemia (presenting as infections) (c) metabolic abnormalities (light chain production and hypercalcaemia) presenting as renal failure with renal amyloid.

This lady presented with back pain due to spinal deposits of plasma cells which had caused partial collapse of the body of the T6 vertebra and subsequent cord compression. This presentation, along with unexplained infections, represents the commonest first clinical manifestation of the disease.

In the initial screening investigations there are usually clues in the haematology and biochemical profile. Almost invariably there is bone marrow suppression with resultant normochromic normocytic anaemia. This may occasionally be leuco-ery-throblastic due to marrow replacement. In addition iron deficiency may occur due to the bleeding tendency. Granulocytopenia is not commonly found at presentation and is usually a later feature as marrow is replaced by abnormal cells or following chemotherapy. The white cells may be functionally abnormal, but this aspect is not routinely tested. Platelets are usually normal in number at presentation but may be functionally abnormal due to the levels of circulating paraprotein. The peripheral blood film usually shows rouleaux formation – the red cells clump together under the influence of the paraproteins, especially at lower temperatures. It is rare for plasma cells to appear in the peripheral blood film. The erythrocyte sedimentation rate is almost always raised (as shown also by the plasma viscosity) and is often well over 100mm in the first hour. In this lady it was surprisingly low at 68mm in the first hour.

An initial biochemical profile is important to establish a baseline for subsequent assessment of renal function and calcium level. Note that correction of the measured calcium is important as the albumin is low at 33g/l.

A range of investigations should immediately lead on from these preliminary screening results and the diagnosis is confirmed if they show two out of the following three: paraproteinaemia, bone marrow plasmacytosis and multiple lytic lesions of bones.

Paraproteins

This lady has a typical serum protein electrophoretic pattern with a dense M-component which is found in about three-quarters of cases. This band is composed of IgG (in 60 per cent of patients), IgA (in about 20 per cent) or light chains only (in about 20 per cent). The other immunoglobulins (IgD,E,M) are rare. This lady had an IgG band.

Paraproteins are best detected in the urine (either neat or concentrated) by immunoelectrophoresis. Bence-Jones protein (i.e. intact immunoglobulin) may be detected by heating the urine gradually – it precipitates at 40°C and redissolves at 60°C.

Levels of β_2-microglobulin should also be measured, as this is associated with class I HLA antigens and the level will give an indication of myeloma mass.

Bone marrow

This is an essential investigation but in severely affected patients there may be difficulty with a 'dry tap' in the sternum. If this occurs, trephine biopsy of the iliac crest is required with 'finger prints' of the core (produced by rolling the biopsy sample on a microscope slide) and histology. In this patient the marrow was hypercellular on aspiration and showed diagnostic features, i.e. an excess of plasma cells (>20 per cent of cells). Typical abnormal plasma cells are shown in Figs 6 & 7. Associated Russell bodies are seen in many of these cells – these are rounded globules of IgG at the edge of the cytoplasm.

Radiology

X-ray of the skeleton is important as erosion of bone is a common finding. The X-ray of the thoracic spine (Fig. 1) showed partial collapse of T6 with destruction of the spinal pedicles. Pathological fractures of this type are a characteristic and common feature. Other bones which should be X-rayed include the skull, pelvis and long bones. The characteristic features are multiple punched out lytic lesions with generalized demineralization. The lesions are only rarely osteosclerotic (<1 per cent).

Prognosis

The prognosis in multiple myeloma is poor despite treatment, with a median survival time of about 2 years in the older patients and only marginally longer in younger people.

CASE 13:

A Contraindication to Thrombolysis in Acute Myocardial Infarction

A 40-year-old man was admitted as an emergency with a 2 hour history of severe crushing central chest pain. He was a heavy cigarette smoker and admitted to drinking alcohol to great excess (conservatively estimated at more than 100 units per week). Both his parents had died of ischaemic heart disease in their 50s. His past medical history included a story over many years of vague 'indigestion, heartburn and waterbrash' for which he had never been investigated and for which he took an occasional teaspoonful of baking soda.

Question 1: What is the differential diagnosis of the acute presentation?

Answer: Myocardial infarction
Unstable angina
Pericarditis
Pancreatitis
Aortic dissection
Perforated duodenal ulcer
Pulmonary embolus

Question 2: Fig. 1 is the ECG taken in the Emergency Department. What does it show?

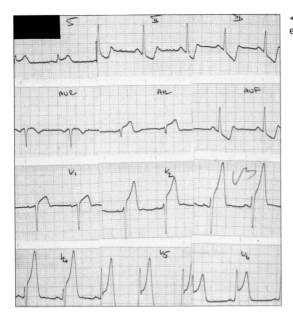

◀ **1** ECG on arrival at hospital emergency room.

Answer: Sinus rhythm. ST elevation in leads I, aVL, V1–V6. Reciprocal ST depression in leads II, III, and aVF. The appearances are consistent with acute anterior myocardial infarction.

Question 3: Describe the immediate management of this patient.

Answer: Administer aspirin (150mg p.o. stat), establish venous access and leave a cannula *in situ*, administer high-flow oxygen by mask, relieve pain with opiate, attach to cardiac monitor. Transfer to coronary care unit for thrombolysis or, if there is a delay in transfer, start thrombolysis in emergency room, if there are no contraindications.

Question 4: What contraindications should be considered before starting thrombolysis?

Answer: The major contraindications to thrombolysis are summarized in **Table 1**.

Table 1 Contraindications to the use of thrombolytic therapy.

Active internal bleeding (from peptic ulcer, ulcerative colitis, haemorrhagic strokes, etc.)
Recent major surgery
Parturition
Recent liver or kidney biopsy
Recent arterial puncture
Trauma or fractures
Recent cardiopulmonary resuscitation (if any possibility of resulting rib fractures or organ damage)
Uncontrolled hypertension
Infective endocarditis
Diabetic retinopathy
Coagulation factor defect
Thrombocytopenia
Other known bleeding disorder

Shortly after arrival in the coronary care unit the patient started vomiting coffee-ground material and he then brought up 200ml of fresh blood. This haematemesis was associated with a fall in BP to 110/60 mmHg and a pulse rate of 96/min.

Question 5: How does this influence his treatment?

Answer: The haematemesis is an absolute contraindication to thrombolytic therapy. This new complication was managed by colloid infusion (plasma protein substitute) and later by the transfusion of cross matched blood to maintain his pulse rate below 100/min and his blood pressure above 100 mmHg. Urine output was monitored. An H_2 blocker was given intravenously to reduce acid output in the stomach.

Case 13

Question 6: As thrombolytic therapy is contraindicated what alternative methods to restore blood flow in the affected coronary artery should be considered?

Answer: (1) Immediate coronary artery bypass grafting.
(2) Immediate coronary angioplasty.

In this case it was decided that the ECG appearances suggested that he would have a haemodynamically significant myocardial infarction if left untreated. Immediate coronary artery bypass grafting is a major procedure which can only be undertaken after definition of the lesion by coronary angiography, and, like thrombolysis, it is contraindicated by the presence of an actively bleeding lesion elsewhere. The patient was therefore taken for coronary angiography with a view to angioplasty.

Fig. 2 is the initial coronary angiogram.

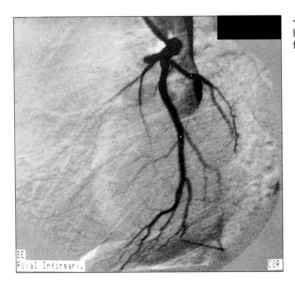

◀ **2** Coronary angiogram (left lateral projection) – freeze frame from first cine run.

Question 7: Which coronary artery is occluded? (If you are uncertain about coronary angiographic anatomy, the ECG findings should give you a clue).

Answer: The left anterior descending coronary artery is occluded proximally. Only a stump is visible.

Angioplasty was undertaken and the post-angioplasty angiogram is shown in Fig. 3.

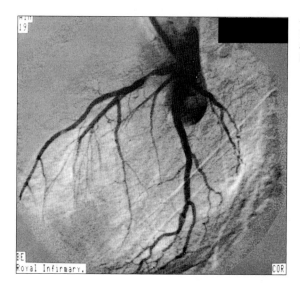

◀**3** Coronary angiogram (left lateral projection) obtained after angioplasty. Compare with Fig. 2.

Question 8: **What is the result of the angioplasty?**

Answer: There is now good perfusion of the left anterior descending artery. However, a residual stenosis remains. This can, if necessary, be dealt with electively after a period of stabilization.

Three days later the patient was endoscoped to determine the site of bleeding and the abnormal finding is shown in the view of the gastric antrum in Fig. 4.

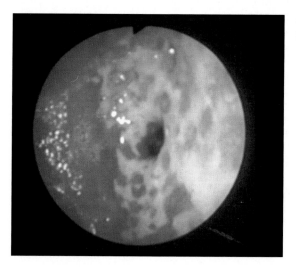

◀**4** Endoscopic view of the gastric antrum.

Case 13

Question 9: What is shown here?

Answer: The patient has severe antral gastritis. No blood clots or other signs of recent bleeding are seen in this view, but the tissue was friable, and it bled easily when touched with the endoscope.

Question 10: As it is important that he continues to take his aspirin to prevent re-thrombosis at the site of angioplasty what additional drug should be taken concomitantly to aid healing of the gastritis and protect the gastric mucosa from the effects of aspirin?

Answer: Misoprostol can be given. This is an analogue of the naturally occurring prostaglandin E_1 and has been shown to protect the gastroduodenal mucosa by inhibiting basal, stimulated and nocturnal acid secretion; it also reduces the proteolytic activity of the gastric fluid and increases the bicarbonate and mucus secretion. An H_2-receptor antagonist should probably also be continued for at least the period of his admission to hospital.

COMMENT

Thrombolytic therapy is now agreed to be a highly effective treatment for acute coronary occlusion with myocardial infarction. Its use should be routine in patients who reach medical attention within 4 hours of the onset of symptoms, but it is contraindicated in some patients. Percutaneous transluminal coronary angioplasty (PTCA) provides an alternative mode of therapy in many of these patients. While it is a well-established technique for the treatment of chronic stable angina, however, angioplasty has yet to be shown to have a defined role in the routine treatment of acute coronary occlusion. Most studies suggest that early angioplasty following thrombolytic therapy in acute myocardial infarction confers no benefit over a policy of delayed intervention. However immediate angioplasty without prior thrombolytic therapy has been shown to be safe and may be highly effective. This should certainly be considered in a case, such as this, when there is clear evidence of a potentially large myocardial infarction but an absolute contraindication to thrombolytic therapy.

If the patient were to have further chest pain during convalescence or to develop objective signs of on-going myocardial ischaemia repeat angioplasty to this lesion should be considered.

His gastritis should be kept under review, and its full healing confirmed by repeat endoscopy. Biopsy of the gastric antrum with urease testing, microscopy and culture for *Helicobacter pylori* infection, followed by appropriate combination therapy, is indicated if the gastritis persists or recurs.

A major effort must be made to control the patient's other risk factors for coronary artery disease, namely smoking, hyperlipidaemia (total cholesterol was 7.4 mmol/l) and obesity. His alcoholic excess may be helped by appropriate counselling.

CASE 14:
An Obese Woman Admitted with Chest Pain

This 48-year-old postmenopausal woman was admitted under the influence of alcohol about an hour after suffering a 10 minute episode of central chest pain, which was precipitated by the exertion of performing at a 'karaoke' night out. She had a 2 year history of hypertension which had been treated by her family doctor with atenolol and a thiazide diuretic. She was not taking any other drug therapy. She had a long history of depression and was also a heavy smoker. As the character of the pain suggested ischaemic heart disease an ECG was performed and blood sent for measurement of creatine kinase levels. Both were found to be normal on each of 3 occasions. The appearance of the patient is shown in Figs 1–4.

Question 1: What features are present in these clinical pictures?

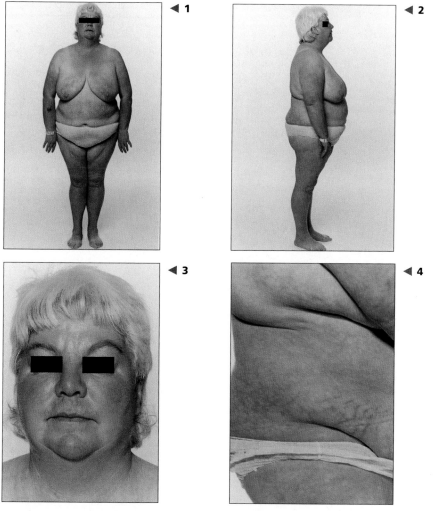

1–4 The patient photographed soon after her admission for investigation.

Case 14

Answer: (a) Gross central obesity
(b) Facial plethora
(c) Facial hirsutism
(d) Purple striae on abdomen, breasts and upper arms.

In addition her blood pressure was 195/100 mmHg but she had no proximal muscle weakness or wasting. The skin was normal and she had no abnormal bruising. Her body mass index was 33.

Question 2: What is the differential diagnosis and what investigations are required?

Answer: (a) Simple obesity with hypertension and ischaemic heart disease
(b) Cushing's syndrome
(c) Pseudo-Cushing's Syndrome

Required investigations include:

Haematology	Haemoglobin	13.4g/dl
	Haematocrit	0.393
	MCV	105fl
	MCH	30.6pg
	MCHC	34.2g/dl
	WBC	$7.2 \times 10^9/l$
	Platelets	$105 \times 10^9/l$
	Film	red cells show macrocytosis
Biochemistry	Creatinine	89μmol/l
	Sodium	136mmol/l
	Potassium	4.1mmol/l
	Bicarbonate	26mmol/l
	Glucose (random)	8.3mmol/l
	Bilirubin	15μmol/l
	Alkaline phosphatase	45u/l
	Albumin	38g/l
	Total cholesterol	8.6mmol/l
	Gamma glutamyl transpeptidase	300μ/l
	Plasma cortisol am	820mmol/l
	pm	657mmol/l
	Urinary free cortisol	450mmol/24 hours
	X-ray chest	Normal

Question 3: Comment on these test results.

Answer: The random blood glucose is suspiciously high, so a fasting sample should be taken. The X-ray of the chest is normal. Note the high MCV, the presence of macrocytes, the lower than normal platelet count and the elevated gamma glutamyl transpeptidase.

The values of plasma cortisol show loss of the diurnal rhythm (the evening value is high) and the urinary free cortisol is elevated.

These results were obtained after a period of stress and their interpretation is difficult. Following the administration of 1mg of dexamethasone (given at midnight) the 9a.m. level of plasma cortisol was 54nmol/l – confirming normal suppression of the pituitary – adrenal axis, and excluding Cushing's syndrome. The diurnal cortisol values were repeated 7 days later and showed

Plasma cortisol a.m.	650nmol/l
p.m.	187nmol/l
Urinary free cortisol	204nmol/24 hours

COMMENT

This lady presented with chest pain which clinically was very suggestive of ischaemic cardiac pain. She had several risk factors for arterial disease; hypertension, smoking habit, obesity and possible glucose intolerance (though this is not confirmed by a single high level in a stressed patient). It also rapidly became clear that she was drinking regularly, far in excess of her declared number of units (25) per week. On initial examination it was suggested that she had Cushing's syndrome, because of her moon face, central obesity, purple striae and hypertension. The initial screening tests were abnormal (plasma cortisol diurnal rhythm and urinary free cortisols). Dexamethasone suppression testing with 1mg showed adrenal suppression. Repeat testing after 7 days of alcohol withdrawal confirmed the diagnosis of pseudo-Cushing's syndrome induced by alcohol.

The high MCV and the low platelet count are characteristic of the alcoholic and this is also reflected in the elevated gamma-GT level. The cause of the macrocytosis is probably a combination of folate deficiency and a direct effect of alcohol (or its metabolite) on the red cell membrane. Similarly thrombocytopenia is related to folate deficiency and a direct effect of alcohol on maturation of megakaryocytes in the marrow.

This lady was persuaded to stop drinking and control her calorie intake. This rapidly produced improvement in her haematological and biochemical indices and a downward trend in her weight and blood pressure.

Alcoholic pseudo-Cushing's should be borne in mind in the differential diagnosis of hypercortisolaemia. Typically, there is loss of diurnal variation of cortisol and increased urinary excretion of cortisol, with many clinical features of Cushing's syndrome. There may be failure to suppress 9a.m. cortisol after overnight dexamethasone, and in this situation, alcoholic pseudo-Cushing's can be differentiated by a normal cortisol rise in response to insulin-induced hypoglycaemia – this rise in cortisol is lost in Cushing's syndrome. Hypoglycaemia would have been dangerous in this lady, who has ischaemic heart disease, and the diagnosis was reached by demonstrating return of the control of cortisol secretion to normal following withdrawal from alcohol.

CASE 15:
Sudden Onset of Facial Palsy

This 72-year-old woman was admitted because of the sudden onset of a facial palsy, which had presented with clumsiness on chewing and dribbling of fluids from the corner of her mouth. The progress of the weakness was rapid and within 24 hours it had produced the appearances shown in Figs 1a & 1b. The patient had been generally unwell with a pyrexia for the previous few days.

Question 1: What typical features are shown in Figs 1a & 1b.

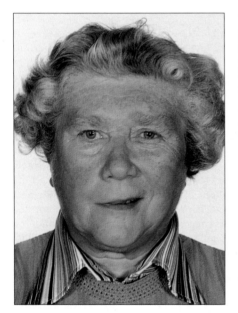

▲ **1a** The patient has been asked to smile.

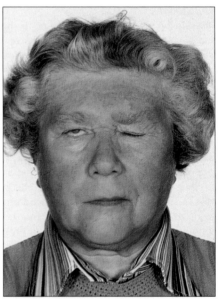

▲ **1b** The patient has been asked to close her eyes tightly.

Answer: In **Fig. 1a** she has been asked to smile. Note the weakness of the right facial muscles, which results in an unfurrowed forehead on the right and a failure of elevation of the right side of the month. In **Fig. 1b** she has been asked to close her eyes, but this is not possible on the affected side. In this patient, as commonly, the resting facial appearance was nearly normal.

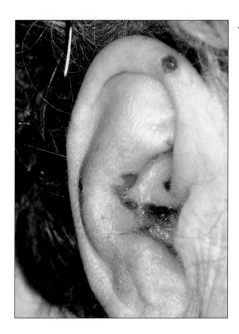

◀ **2** The patient's right ear.

In addition to the above history the patient complained of pain in her right ear. Examination of the external ear showed the appearances seen in Fig. 2.

Question 2: Describe the appearances. What disease is this?

Answer: There are multiple vesicles in the external auditory meatus and on the pinna. Some of the lesions have burst and early scab formation is present.
This is the typical manifestation of herpes zoster infection of the geniculate ganglion of the 7th nerve (Ramsay Hunt syndrome).

Question 3: Where else should the clinician look for signs?

Answer: Unilateral vesicular lesions may be found in the auditory canal and on the tongue (**Fig. 3**), palate and pharynx. In addition, taste may be affected and formal testing of taste should be carried out on the anterior two-thirds of the tongue. Occasionally the 8th nerve is also involved with resultant impairment of hearing.

Case 15

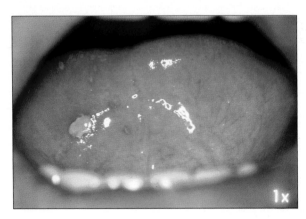

3 The patient's tongue. Multiple vesicles, which burst and ulcerate, are seen on the right side of the under surface.

1x

Question 4: What treatment may shorten the course of this painful condition?

Answer: Acyclovir, given early in the course of the disease, has been shown to reduce the duration of the infection and the resulting nerve involvement.

Question 5: What ophthalmological complication may occur and how can it be prevented?

Answer: Keratitis may result from inability to close the eye on the affected side. Frequent instillation of moisturizing drops or even temporary tarsorrhaphy may be necessary to prevent corneal damage.

Question 6: What is the prognosis?

Answer: The prognosis for full recovery is excellent in the Ramsay Hunt syndrome (as in Bell's palsy, where the underlying cause of the 7th nerve palsy is unknown). Permanent nerve damage or muscle weakness is rare, but post-herpetic neuralgia may occur.

COMMENT

Geniculate herpes zoster (Ramsay Hunt syndrome) is a relatively rare presentation of herpes zoster (shingles) which may be expected to be seen in 4 per 1000 patients registered in a British general practice per year. The infecting agent is the *Varicella zoster* virus which may have been present in the geniculate ganglion for many years or may represent a new infection. As with herpes zoster elsewhere, reactivation of the latent virus may occur in sensory root ganglia in the elderly and in those who are immunocompromised by HIV infection, lymphoma, other malignant disease, steroid therapy, diabetes mellitus or following chemo- and radiotherapy. Unlike chickenpox, the other manifestation of *Varicella zoster* virus infection, there is no seasonal variation in incidence.

The usual clinical manifestations are a few days of malaise and pyrexia followed by the first local manifestations such as severe pain in the ear and a localized rash in the external auditory meatus (Fig. 2) and on the surrounding ear. The rash starts as vesicles, becomes pustular and scabs over to heal with scarring. Additional examination may show the typical lesions on the tympanic membrane and on the palate, tongue (Fig. 3) and pharynx. This is accompanied by an ipsilateral lower motor neurone lesion of the facial nerve (Fig. 1) and associated with loss of taste in the anterior two-thirds of the tongue. The 8th nerve may also be affected in which case there may be hyperacusis, vertigo and occasionally hearing loss. Healing with some local scarring is usually complete in 2–3 weeks but may be followed by persisting pain (post-herpetic neuralgia). In the majority of cases the lower motor neurone palsy recovers fully in 2–3 weeks.

The diagnosis is usually obvious clinically but the presence of virus may be shown by culture of vesicle fluid, by direct EM or by fluorescent antibody staining.

Administration of acyclovir at the first manifestation has been shown to shorten the course of the disease.

CASE 16:

Muscle Weakness, Fits and Dark Urine

A 21-year-old male student was referred to an out patient clinic with a history of apparent intermittent painless haematuria, which had been preceded by unconsciousness.

Further questioning about the period of preceding unconsciousness suggested the possibility of an epileptiform seizure; it had come on with no warning, the patient had bitten his tongue, had been incontinent of urine and had bruised himself on falling. He had then been unconscious on the floor for several minutes. As this episode was not witnessed it was not possible to say if he had had tonic–clonic movements.

There was no history of urinary tract infections, of renal colic or of passing a calculus. He denied any recent trauma. The only past medical history of note was a chronic complaint of weakness, stiffness and cramping pain in the muscles, especially in the legs, but also occasionally in the arms and even the jaw. This effect was produced by exertion and relieved by rest, and had occurred for as long as the patient could remember.

On examination he appeared fit and well, there was no muscle weakness or wasting, no neurological abnormality and no evidence of limb ischaemia. Abdominal examination was unremarkable.

Question 1: What initial investigations should be done?

Answer: The following tests were done:

Haematology	Haemoglobin	13g/dl
	PCV	0.395
	MCV	78.5fl
	MCH	25.8pg
	MCHC	32.8g/dl
	WBC	$5.5 \times 10^9/l$
	Platelets	$259 \times 10^9/l$
	ESR	6mm in 1st hour
	Blood film	Normal
Biochemistry	Sodium	141mmol/l
	Potassium	4.2mmol/l
	Chloride	98mmol/l
	Urea	4.2mmol/l
	Creatinine	80µmol/l

Urine
Chemical and microscopic examination of the urine was entirely normal, and no red cells, white cells or casts were present. Culture was also negative.

EEG	This is shown in **Fig. 1**

Question 2: What diagnostic abnormalities are present in the EEG (Fig. 1)?

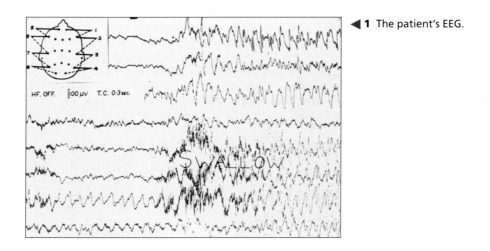

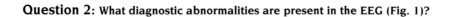

1 The patient's EEG.

Answer: This shows occasional paroxysmal bursts of sharp waves and spikes and slow waves suggestive of tonic clonic (grand mal) epilepsy.

While under investigation he had another fit and after this developed dark urine as shown in Fig. 2.

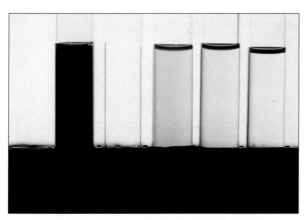

◀ 2 The patient's dark urine (left) compared with urine samples from other individuals.

Question 3: What may this urine colour be due to?

Answer: Brown coloured urine is most often due to the presence of red blood cells, but substances including haemoglobin, myoglobin, porphyrin and melanin, as well as ingested colourings such as beetroot, aniline dye (from sweets) and phenolic drugs, can also result in pigmented urine.

Case 16

This sample reacted positively for blood using conventional strip tests. These strip tests depend on the peroxidase properties of the haem ring of haemoglobin which, in the presence of peroxide, oxidizes *o*-toluidine to a blue colour. The reaction is also catalysed by myoglobin. The presence of myoglobin in the urine of this patient was confirmed by spectroscopy, polyacrylamide gel electrophoresis and immunodiffusion techniques.

The creatine kinase (CK) level was measured on this occasion and found to be 16,400u/l. This was thought initially to reflect the recent tonic–clonic epileptiform seizure and the CK levels were accordingly followed over several days. The value fell to a plateau of about 1100u/l.

Question 4: What is the likely diagnosis?

Answer: McArdle's disease (Type V glycogen storage disease of muscle due to phosphorylase deficiency).

Question 5: What additional tests should be done?

Answer: a) Glucagon stimulation test
b) Ischaemic lactate test
c) Electromyography
d) Muscle biopsy

Results

(a) A glucagon stimulation test gave the following results after 1mg of glucagon was given intramuscularly at time zero.

Time (min)	Blood glucose (mmol/l)
0	4.6
5	6.5
15	7.6
25	7.5

Glucagon stimulates the release of glucose from liver glycogen stores but has no effect on muscle glycogen. This is a normal test result, confirming that glycogenolysis is occurring normally in his liver.

(b) An ischaemic lactate test was carried out using a sphygmomanometer cuff placed around the upper arm and inflated above the systolic pressure. The subject then exercised the hand by squeezing the sphygmomanometer bulb once every second for a minute at which time the cuff was released. Absence of a rise in blood lactate under these conditions is a characteristic of all diseases where there is impairment in the conversion of glycogen or glucose to lactate in striated muscle. This includes deficiencies in muscle phosphorylase, phosphorylase-b-kinase, amylo-l,6-glucosidase, glucose phosphate isomerase, phosphofructokin-ase-l or other glycolytic enzymes.

In this case the following results were obtained:

Blood lactate (mmol/l) before and after ischaemic exercise:

	Before	After
Patient	1.6	1.9
Control	1.1	4.2

This patient did not show a rise in blood lactate concentration after ischaemic exercise. This positive test is an indication for muscle biopsy to enable histochemical or biochemical analysis of the activities of the various muscle enzymes listed above.

(c) Electromyography demonstrated normal muscle contraction as compared to a healthy control but a long delay in recovery.

(d) A muscle biopsy was performed on the left gastrocnemius muscle. Histology of this sample showed characteristic changes of McArdle's disease, i.e. vacuolation of muscle fibres (Fig. 3), many vacuoles giving a positive reaction with specific stains for glycogen. Histochemistry of this sample demonstrated a complete absence of muscle phosphorylase activity (Figs 4 & 5) and four times the normal amount of glycogen. This is diagnostic of McArdle's disease.

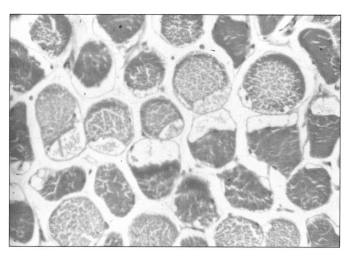

◀ **3** Vacuolation of striated muscle fibres is a characteristic finding in McArdle's disease (H & E section).

Case 16

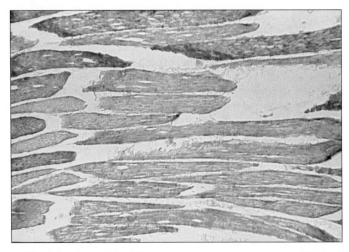

◀ **4** Muscle from a normal individual stained for muscle phosphorylase activity – a normal result.

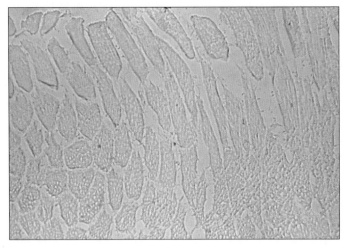

◀ **5** Muscle from the patient, stained for muscle phosphorylase activity. The pale staining reflects the complete absence of muscle phosphorylase.

Question 6: What is the inheritance of this disease?

Answer: McArdle's disease usually follows an autosomal recessive mode of inheritance. In agreement with this, investigation of this family (**Fig. 6**) demonstrated the parents and two of the patient's siblings to be clinically unaffected, and to show a normal lactate response to ischaemic exercise. Three more of the patient's siblings, one female and two male, complained of muscle pains in their legs, but not for other muscle groups, on exercise. None of the siblings had experienced myoglobinuria nor did any of them give a history of episodes of unconsciousness. The three siblings that complained of muscle cramps all failed to show an increase in blood lactate on ischaemic exercise and were considered to be affected by McArdle's disease, although to a lesser extent than the index case.

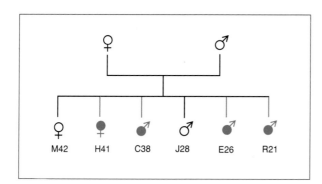

◄ **6** The patient's family tree. The patient is R (age 21). Other affected family members are indicated in blue.

M42   H41   C38   J28   E26   R21

COMMENT

The combination of muscle pain and weakness on exercise with myoglobinuria points very strongly to a disease primarily of voluntary muscle. The common causes of myoglobinuria are widespread crush injury to muscle or localized ischaemic muscle necrosis. This patient's history eliminated these two possibilities. Polymyositis and glycogen storage diseases may also cause myoglobinuria. The rare syndrome of paroxysmal myoglobinuria, or rhabdomyolysis of unknown aetiology, where patients suffer acute attacks of severe cramp-like muscle pain and tenderness associated with weakness or paralysis and accompanied by profuse myoglobinuria, is thought to be due to carnitine palmityl transferase deficiency.

Although these diseases are rare they should be considered in a case with such specific muscle symptoms. Specific glycogen storage disease of muscle is usually fairly benign in nature and presents with exercise-induced muscle pain, cramps and myoglobinuria. McArdle's disease (myophosphorylase deficiency), Tarui's disease (muscle phosphofructokinase deficiency), Di Mauro's disease (muscle phosphoglycerate-mutase or phosphoglycerate-kinase deficiency) and muscle lactate dehydrogenase deficiency are all included in this group.

Case 16

Patients with McArdle's disease (Type V glycogen storage disease, muscle phosphorylase deficiency) typically present in early adult life with muscle pains, stiffness and cramps associated with the passage of dark brown urine (myoglobinuria). The myoglobin in the urine results from muscle damage. It gives a positive orthotoluidine test (as does haemoglobin) and it should be differentiated by polyacrylamide gel electrophoresis or by immunodiffusion where confusion is possible. The metabolic defect is the absence of skeletal muscle glycogen phosphorylase but, surprisingly, this produces few symptoms during childhood. The disease usually presents in the 2nd or 3rd decade of life with severe muscle cramps and secondary myoglobinuria. There was a history of long standing muscle weakness especially after exercise and eventually clinical evidence of proximal muscle wasting. A spectrum of biochemical abnormalities was also present. Muscle enzymes in serum were elevated due to leakage from muscle cells during exertion. These included creatine phosphokinase (CK), lactate dehydrogenase (LDH) and aldolase (AH). The blood sugar level was normal and hypoglycaemia was not found after exertion.

Screening tests for muscle glycogenolysis include measurement of the lactate content of venous blood of a limb after ischaemic exercising (there is no rise when there is a failure of muscle glycogenolysis) and measurement of the blood glucose after stimulation with glucagon (the glucose level rises when there is normal glycogenolysis in the liver). The block in ATP formation by anaerobic glycolysis diminishes the availability of high-energy phosphate, and thus interferes with function, causes leakage of cell contents from the damaged membrane and hence myoglobinuria. Continued injury following exercise results in muscle cell death and subsequent muscle atrophy.

This patient also had epileptic fits, which have been described in about 5 per cent of patients. The cause is not known, but treatment was started in this man using sodium valproate.

McArdle's disease is inherited as an autosomal recessive, as shown in the family tree (Fig. 4). The disease may be screened for by measurement of muscle enzymes, especially after exercise, and confirmed by muscle biopsy.

The disease usually runs a benign course but severe exercise should be avoided. Minor muscle wasting may be the only clinical consequence. A similar clinical presentation to McArdle's disease may be found in patients subsequently shown to have phosphofructokinase deficiency. In addition acute alcoholic myopathy may be seen in the chronic alcoholic after an acute drinking episode, the clinical presentation being with muscle pain, tenderness and myoglobinuria. Such patients may also have an acquired deficiency of muscle phosphorylase.

CASE 17:

A 38-Year-Old Man with Palpitations

A 38-year-old man presented to the Accident and Emergency Department with a 12 hour history of palpitations These took the form of an awareness of his heart beating too rapidly to count. He felt sweaty and breathless but there were no other associated symptoms. He had given a history of palpitations since childhood. These had occurred infrequently over the past 10 years but had never lasted for as long as this episode. Over the years he had learned various ways to stop his palpitations but none had worked on this occasion.

There was no other significant past medical history, he was a non-smoker, denied excessive alcohol intake and was on no drug therapy.

On examination he looked pale and was sweating. The pulse rate was in excess of 200 per minute. Blood pressure was 100/60mmHg. Heart sounds were normal and there were no signs of cardiac failure. The rest of the physical examination was normal.

Question 1: Fig. 1 is his 12-lead ECG on arrival at hospital. What does it show?

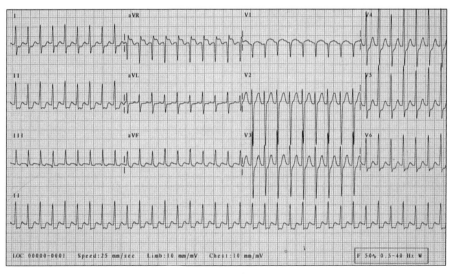

▲ **1** The patient's 12-lead ECG on arrival at hospital.

Answer: A rapid narrow-complex tachycardia with a rate of approximately 220 per minute.

Case 17

Question 2: What is the likely diagnosis?

Answer: Paroxysmal supraventricular tachycardia, probably due to AV nodal re-entry.

Question 3: What bedside clinical test might help establish the diagnosis?

Answer: Carotid sinus massage may terminate the arrhythmia.

Question 4: How is this carried out?

Answer: Locate the carotid pulse and rub the carotid in a circular motion for up to 10 seconds. Do this only on one side at a time but, if necessary, try each side in turn.

He knew of several other manoeuvres which he had used to terminate his own attacks in the past.

Question 5: What might they be and what is their mechanism of action?

Answer: Straining against a closed glottis, i.e. the Valsalva manoeuvre; sticking his fingers down his throat; pressing hard on an eyeball; swallowing crushed ice; dipping his head in cold water (the diving reflex). These, like carotid sinus massage, all stimulate the vagus nerve which increases AV nodal delay and may interrupt the re-entry circuit responsible for continuation of the arrhythmia.

Lead II ECG monitoring was set up and he was given a drug by rapid intravenous bolus at point A with almost immediate effect (Fig. 2).

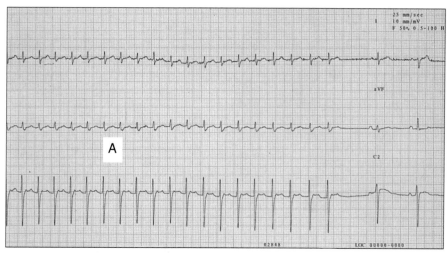

▲ 2 The effect of a rapid IV drug bolus on the arrhythmia.

Question 6: What two drugs may be used to terminate such arrhythmias?

Answer: Adenosine and verapamil. In this case 3mg of adenosine was given by intravenous bolus.

COMMENT

Paroxysmal supraventricular tachycardia is the clinical term used for a variety of arrhythmias arising from the atria. In this case a more correct term is AV nodal re-entry tachycardia, in which there are dual pathways between the atria and ventricles either within or around the AV node.

The simplest form of treatment for an acute attack is to carry out vagal stimulation by the Valsalva manoeuvre or other manoeuvres which patients can be taught to carry out. In this case the attack could not be terminated by this means, and the patient was admitted for pharmacological or electrical cardioversion. Intravenous adenosine or verapamil are the drugs of choice to terminate these acute episodes but verapamil must be used with caution in patients taking a beta blocker. Occasionally DC cardioversion or overdrive pacing is necessary to terminate the arrhythmia.

Prophylactic therapy is indicated if the arrhythmias occur frequently or are symptomatically very troublesome. Verapamil, flecainide, propafenone, disopyramide, digoxin and beta blockers can all be used. Amiodarone may also be effective but should be used only for the most refractory arrhythmias due to its long term toxic effects. If the arrhythmia does not respond to treatment or there are side effects from the drug therapy other options to consider are an anti-tachycardia pacemaker or mapping and ablation of the aberrant pathway. Radio-frequency catheter ablation is being increasingly used in this situation with considerable success.

CASE 18:

Breathlessness, Unproductive Cough and Weight Loss

A 32-year-old woman was admitted at the request of her family doctor with suspected acute pneumonia. Over the past 5 months she had been 'off colour', with anorexia, nausea and gradual but progressive weight loss of about 14kg to her present weight of 52kg. She also complained of intermittent nocturnal fever, and had become progressively short of breath. She was now breathless on minor exertion, and she had an irritating non-productive cough. For the 2 days prior to this admission she had had a niggling left shoulder tip and subcostal pain which was pleuritic in nature and had become more severe and localized in the few hours prior to admission.

Her past history included an ectopic pregnancy 12 years ago, a termination of pregnancy 6 years ago and a surgical admission for lower abdominal pain 2 years ago, during which time investigations had shown positive anti-mitochondrial antibody (but this was not further investigated). No cause was found for her abdominal pain, which was ascribed to 'pelvic inflammation'. She had also been seen by her GP about $2^1/_2$ years ago with a maculo-papular rash attributed to amoxycillin allergy (Fig. 1).

She smoked 20 cigarettes per day, kept no pets and was a divorced full time housewife who looked after two children. Prior to this admission she had been given two courses of antibiotics (erythromycin and a cephalosporin) but these had not helped her symptoms of weight loss and breathlessness.

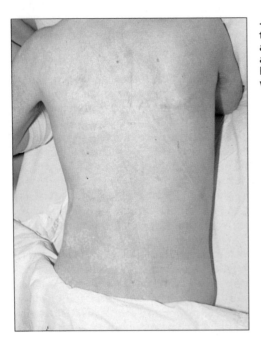

◄ **1** A maculo-papular rash similar to that which occurred $2^1/_2$ years before admission, and which was ascribed to amoxycillin 'allergy'. The amoxycillin had been prescribed for a sore throat with local lymph node enlargement.

Question 1: What conditions must be considered in the differential diagnosis of her weight loss?

Answer:

(a) Diabetes mellitus and thyrotoxicosis had both been thought of by the GP who had measured her fasting blood sugar (4.6mmol/l) despite a negative history of polyuria, polydipsia and thirst. She had developed oral and vaginal thrush following antibiotic therapy, which were treated with amphotericin B oral lozenges and nystatin pessaries. In addition, despite there being no other symptoms or signs of thyrotoxicosis, the GP had measured the T4 level, which was 117nmol/l, and the TSH, 1.36mU/l.

(b) Tuberculosis – there was no family history, she had been given BCG vaccination at school and was known from the medical records to have subsequently been Mantoux positive. There was no history of any positive contacts among friends or family.

(c) Malignancy – lymphoma had been considered as a possibility but no pathologically enlarged lymph nodes were palpable, the spleen was not palpable and no skin nodules were present. There were no signs to suggest other underlying malignancy.

(d) Malabsorption syndromes – there were no symptoms referrable to the alimentary system to support this diagnosis (though she had recently been constipated). There had only been one episode of severe diarrhoea while she was on a Spanish holiday the previous year and this had resolved following antibiotic therapy from a local doctor.

(e) Infective endocarditis is a possible explanation for her symptoms, although she gave no history of valvular heart disease, and there were no suggestive signs on examination.

(f) AIDS is a recognized cause of weight loss, especially in Africa and Asia, but also in the UK, and the possibility should be considered in this patient.

Examination of the patient confirmed that she had a fever (38.5°C). There was slight central cyanosis. Her tongue was rather sore and raw and had been since her last course of antibiotics; this had persisted despite the recent use of amphotericin B (Fig. 2). There was no lymphadenopathy and her skin and joints were normal. Examination of the chest showed some local tenderness over the lower left anterior chest wall and there was a zone of coarse crepitations in the left axilla.

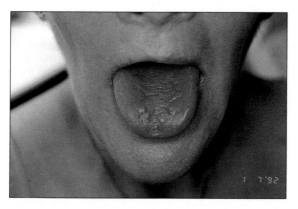

◀ **2** The patient had a raw, sore tongue despite the recent use of amphotericin B lozenges.

Case 18

Question 2: What initial investigations should be done?

Answer:

Haematology	Haemoglobin	8.5g/dl
	WBC	$2.4 \times 10^9/l$
	Platelets	$284 \times 10^9/l$
	Blood film	Red cells normochromic, normocytic
		Lymphopenia and rouleaux formation
	ESR	135mm in 1st hour
	C-reactive protein	100mg/l
Serum Biochemistry	Sodium	136mmol/l
	Potassium	3.8mmol/l
	Urea	4.6mmol/l
	Glucose	6.1mmol/l
	ALT	12u/l
Chest X-ray	This is shown in **Fig. 3**	

Question 3: What does the X-ray of chest (Fig. 3) show?

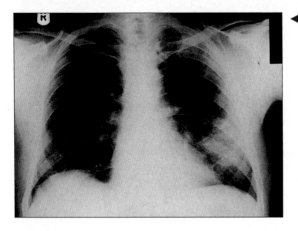

◀ **3** The chest X-ray on admission.

Answer: There is an area of consolidation at the left lower zone which is consistent with pneumonic consolidation.

Question 4: Comment on the haematology/biochemistry results.

Answer: This lady has a severe anaemia which is normochromic and normocytic. The white cell count is low and there is a very low lymphocyte count. The ESR is grossly elevated and this is also reflected in the presence of rouleaux formation on the film. The CRP is also elevated. The biochemical profile gives no clues to the cause of the weight loss.

Question 5: What additional special investigations are urgently required?

Answer:

Arterial Blood Gases	PaO$_2$	7kPa (52mmHg)
	PaCO$_2$	5kPa (38mmHg)
	H$^+$	37nmol/l (pH7.37)
	Standard HCO$_3$	21mmol/l

Pulmonary Function Tests

FEV$_1$/FVC	72% (of predicted for age + size)
PEF	51% of predicted
Dco (diffusing capacity carbon monoxide)	52% of predicted

Microbiology

Serology	Titres for	Legionella	Negative
		Mycoplasma	Negative
		Psittacosis	Negative
		Influenza A & B	Negative
		Adenovirus	Negative

| Sputum | Direct smear of sputum stained by Gram method is shown (**Fig. 4**) |

| Blood culture | +ve *Streptococcus pneumoniae* |

| Mid-stream specimen of urine | Contaminated with *Candida albicans* |

Antinuclear antibodies	Negative
Antimitochondrial antibodies	Negative
Anti smooth muscle antibodies	Negative
Rheumatoid arthritis (Latex)	Negative
Immune complexes	17mg/dl (normal <6mg/dl)

Haematology

Reticulocyte count	<1%
Haptoglobins	Normal
Direct Coombs' test	Positive
Urinary urobilinogen	Negative
Serum iron	14µmol/l
Transferrin	62µmol/l
Saturation	22%
Vit B$_{12}$	925ng/l
Folate	4.8µmol/l

Case 18

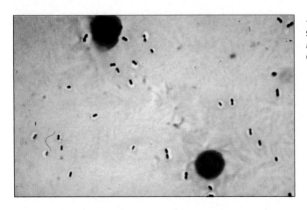

◀ **4** Direct smear of sputum, showing *Streptococcus pneumoniae*. The capsules of the diplococci are clearly seen.

Question 6: What may be deduced from this profile of investigations?

Answer: This patient is severely anoxic with a mixed obstructive/restrictive defect and a marked reduction in transfer factor. Direct smear of the sputum shows the presence of *S. pneumoniae* which also showed in her blood culture. The history, blood gases and respiratory function suggest a more chronic and diffuse cause than the acute onset pneumococcal pneumonia.

The haematology results suggest anaemia of chronic disease. Despite the positive Coombs' test serology there is no other evidence of haemolysis.

Question 7: What additional respiratory tests are required to further define her disease?

Answer: Bronchoscopy with bronchial lavage and biopsy will allow direct investigation of the lung infection.

The specimen from her bronchial lavage is shown in Fig. 5. This confirms the presence of budding forms of *Candida albicans*. Lung biopsy (Figs 6 & 7) showed the presence of *Pneumocystis carinii*.

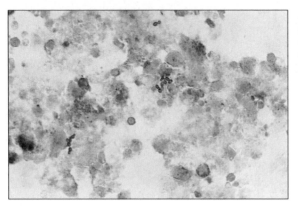

◀ **5** Bronchial lavage sample showing the presence of budding forms of *Candida albicans*.

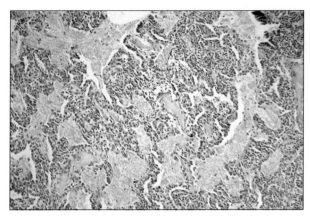

◀ **6** Lung biopsy (H and E stain). The alveoli contain amorphous pink material, and the cellular matter within it is largely composed of *Pneumocystis carinii* cysts. Special staining techniques allow more accurate identification of the trophozoites.

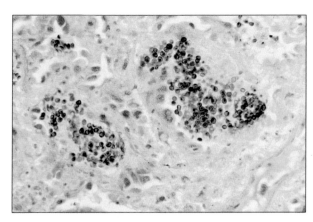

◀ **7** Lung biopsy (Grocott methenamine silver – GMS – stain). Both cysts and trophozoites of *Pneumocystis carinii* are present in large numbers, and some budding forms of *Candida albicans* are also seen.

Question 8: What further test is required?

Answer: Test for HIV antibody. This must be done according to accepted guidelines and must involve prior counselling by a specially trained person. The result of the ELISA HIV antibody test was positive and this was confirmed by the Western blot assay.

Question 9: By what routes could this lady have been infected with HIV virus?

Answer: The commonest route of transmission of HIV infection in the West is still male homosexuality, followed by IV drug abuse (needle sharing), heterosexual inter-course, blood transfusion and transplacental spread (mother to baby). In Africa and the Far East heterosexual spread is the commonest route of transmission. A full list of known routes of transmission appears as **Table 1**.

Case 18

Table 1 Transmission of HIV

Sexual
Homosexual (male)
Bisexual (male)
Heterosexual (male to female, female to male)
Blood
Needle sharing (intravenous drug abusers)
Transfusion of blood and blood products
Organ transplant
Mucous membrane exposure in health care workers
Transmission via needle stick injuries
Transmission via contaminated instruments
Perinatal
Fetus *in utero*
Fetus at delivery

The lady had had blood transfusion following bleeding at an ectopic pregnancy 12 years ago, before routine testing of donor units was routinely done. Record tracing of those donors who had since donated blood was carried out and it was recorded that they had all subsequently tested HIV negative. The episode of sore throat followed by a maculo-papular rash $2^1/_2$ years ago could have represented the sero-conversion phase of her HIV infection, but it could have been the result of an adverse reaction to amoxycillin. Since her divorce she had had several sexual partners and these could not be traced for testing.

Question 10: How would you manage the patient?

Answer: (a) Give oxygen by face mask and maintain it until the pneumonia is successfully treated.

(b) Initiate treatment for *Pneumocystis carinii* with co-trimoxazole (120mg/kg per day in divided doses) and for systemic candidiasis with fluconazole (50mg per day, orally). Corticosteroids have been found to be of value in preventing respiratory failure and mechanical ventilation is indicated when pO_2 <60mmHg(8kPa). Careful monitoring of the arterial blood gases is essential. Anti-retroviral therapy such as zidovudine, can be introduced later.

COMMENT

HIV infection is underdiagnosed, and it may present in almost any field of medical practice much like syphilis did in the last century.

The first manifestation of HIV infection may be an infectious mononucleosis-like illness which may occur 3 weeks to about 3 months after infection. The illness is of sudden onset with attacks of fever, sweating, malaise, myalgia, headache, arthralgia, diarrhoea, lymphadenopathy, and a generalized macular rash more prominent on the trunk. This patient had an episode of illness with a rash which was explained as a skin sensitivity rash to amoxycillin, but as it rapidly cleared it was not pursued further. Its nature cannot be determined in retrospect.

Weight loss is a very common feature of the disease. HIV affects the gut epithelial cells to cause profound malabsorption and its effects may be compounded by various opportunistic infections such as *Cryptosporidium* or *Isospora belli*. This 'slim disease' variant is a common feature of African AIDS, but is less common elsewhere.

This patient's presentation was with acute pneumonia, which was apparently lobar, and a pneumococcus was initially grown from her sputum. Anxiety about her weight loss and her severe hypoxaemia led to further respiratory investigations. Bronchoscopy with bronchial lavage and biopsy showed the presence of *Candida albicans* and of *Pneumocystis carinii*. Testing for HIV antibody was undertaken after obtaining informed consent. This proved to be positive and was confirmed by the Western blot assay. It is likely that the virus was transmitted either sexually or in blood transfused at the time of her ectopic pregnancy 12 years before.

That she was immunocompromised is suggested by the advent of recurrent episodes of candidiasis. Measurement of her CD4 cell count (T-helper lymphocytes) was 0.22×10^9/l and the ratio of CD4:total lymphocyte count ratio was 1:6, confirming immunodeficiency.

The CD4 lymphocyte count is a useful indicator of disease progression. Oral candidiasis is also a strong predictor of both progression and mortality. Other surrogate markers of disease progression include the presence of HIV p24 antigen in the serum and a rising serum concentration of beta 2 microglobulin and neopterin.

With declining cell-mediated immunity opportunistic infections are often the presenting features of the acquired immune deficiency syndrome (AIDS). *Pneumocystis carinii* is the commonest cause of pneumonia, but the latter may also be due to a range of other infections (Table 2).

Table 2 Lung diseases in AIDS

Pneumocystis infection
Bacterial pneumonia
    Streptococcus pneumoniae
    Haemophilus influenzae
    Branhamella catarrhalis
    Staphylococcus aureus
Mycobacterial infection
    Mycobacterium tuberculosis
    Non-tuberculous mycobacteria
    M. avium–intracellulare (terminal phase)
Cytomegalovirus infection
Non-specific interstitial pneumonitis
Lymphocytic interstitial pneumonitis (children)
Kaposi's sarcoma
Bronchial carcinoma

Case 18

For patients in whom *Pneumocystis carinii* pneumonia has been diagnosed the drug of first choice is co-trimoxazole, with pentamidine as the second choice. Following treatment with co-trimoxazole about three-quarters of patients improve as monitored by reduction of the signs and symptoms, reduction of fever, and improvement in oxygenation and in the chest X-ray appearances. Co-trimoxazole must be given IV over 2 hours at a dose of 120mg/kg diluted 1:25 in 5% glucose. This should be given for 14 days and followed by a further week of oral medication at the same dose. At this dose the patient must be monitored carefully for marrow suppression (all elements may be affected), evidence of liver damage and skin rashes.

If there is intolerance to co-trimoxazole then pentamidine should be used by the intravenous route. The dose is 4mg/kg/day, diluted in 250ml of 5% glucose. The side effects of this drug also include marrow suppression as well as renal failure, hypotension, nausea and vomiting and hypoglycaemia.

If co-trimoxazole and pentamidine both fail the options are clindamycin plus primaquine, trimetrexate or eflornithine.

In severe *Pneumocystis carinii* pneumonia, as in this patient, adjuvant cortico-steroids should be started at the same time as specific anti-pneumocystis therapy. As a rule of thumb prednisolone should be given to patients with an arterial oxygen tension ≤9.3kPa or an arterial–alveolar oxygen gradient of ≥4.7kPa. The recommended dose of oral prednisolone is 40mg bd for 5 days followed by 40mg once per day for 5 days then 20mg once per day for 10 days. This regimen will halve the risk of respiratory failure and reduce the risk of death by one-third.

After recovery from *Pneumocystis carinii* pneumonia, prophylaxis should be given and the drug of choice is co-trimoxazole given orally in a dose of 960mg per day. This is usually well tolerated but the patient should be monitored for skin rashes and marrow depression. For patients who are intolerant, nebulized pentamidine (300mg) once every 4 weeks should be given. There is no contraindication to the concomitant use of zidovudine (AZT) during prophylaxis.

CASE 19:
Severe Bruising in a Domestic Assault

A 49-year-old mother was assaulted by her mentally retarded teenage son and beaten with a variety of blunt instruments. She was seen in the Casualty Department because of the extent of the blood loss from multiple lacerations and because of extremely extensive bruising over her whole body (Figs 1–4). She was admitted for observation.

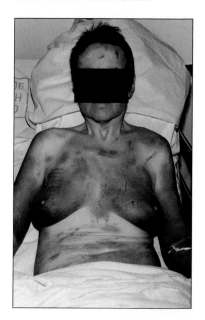
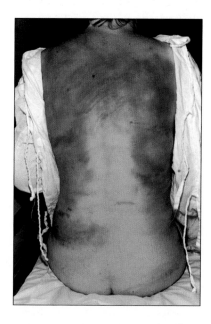
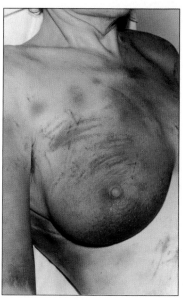
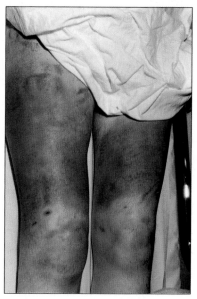

▲ **1–4** The patient had multiple lacerations and extensive bruising over her entire body.

Case 19

She gave a history of a thoracotomy 20 years previously for a cystic tuberculous lung lesion, had received treatment for gastric ulceration 5 years previously and was attending her family doctor for management of sero-negative rheumatoid-type arthritis. Regular medications included ranitidine 150mg bd, Gaviscon, penicillamine 125mg od, naproxen 250mg tds, and paracetamol for analgesia. She had not bothered to take her ranitidine lately, as she was not troubled by any dyspeptic symptoms. Her periods were normal and regular.

The patient was a non-smoker, had no known allergies, but had a strong family history of tuberculosis.

On clinical examination she looked well apart from the extensive bruising, and multiple lacerations. The pulse was 106/min, sinus rhythm; BP 125/70 mm Hg with normal heart sounds and no murmurs. An old right thoracotomy scar was noted and her chest was clinically clear. The abdomen was soft with mild epigastric tenderness, there was no organ enlargement and it was especially noted that there was no splenic enlargement on palpation or percussion. Rectal examination was unremarkable. The patient was fully conscious, alert and orientated, with no focal neurological deficit and had normal reflexes. There was no clinical evidence of any fractures. No active synovitis or arthritis could be detected but there were moderate changes of a symmetrical polyarthritis of the small joints of the hands and feet.

A profile of initial investigations showed the following results:

Haematology	Haemoglobin	5.7g/dl	(The haemoglobin 3 weeks prior to admission was 9.5g/dl)
	MCV	76fl	
	MCH	29.5pg	
	WBC	$7.5 \times 10^9/l$	
	Platelets	$69 \times 10^9/l$	
	ESR	55mm in 1st hour	
Biochemistry	Sodium	143mmol/l	
	Potassium	3.5mmol/l	
	Urea	3.0mmol/l	
	Creatinine	65µmol/l	
Coagulation	Prothrombin time 16sec (control 15sec); APTT = 68sec (control 65sec). Bleeding time (Simplate II method on forearm) 10min.		
Radiology	CXR: Old pleural thickening on right. Old fractures of 8th and 9th ribs. X-rays of skull, spine and long bones showed no fractures.		
Occult blood	Testing for faecal occult blood in stools on three occasions was negative.		

Question 1: What is your interpretation of this data?

Answer: The patient is severely anaemic with a normochromic, normocytic picture. The platelet count is significantly decreased and the screening tests for coagulation disorders are within normal limits. The bleeding time is prolonged and this is in keeping with the low platelet count. The urea and electrolytes are within normal limits. There is no evidence of blood loss from the bowel.

Question 2: What are the probable causes of anaemia in this lady?

Answer:
(i) Gastrointestinal haemorrhage:
95% of gastric ulcers are expected to heal within 3 months on maintenance treatment with H_2 receptor blockers. However, 5% fail to heal on this treatment and are labelled 'resistant' ulcers. Following the withdrawal of maintenance therapy the majority (70-90%) of the ulcers treated with H_2 blockers will relapse and may re-present as haemorrhage without any preceding symptoms. Even in those patients who achieve ulcer remission with H_2 blockers, a proportion (20–30% over 10 years) will relapse. The risk of severe haemorrhage in these patients is very low.
The risk of upper GI haemorrhage from gastric ulcer is substantially increased if the patient is concurrently taking NSAIDs as is the case in this patient.
(ii) Secondary to treatment with penicillamine:
Haematological side effects of penicillamine treatment are well recognized and should be regularly monitored in the out-patient clinic. Most common are agranulocytosis, thrombocytopenia or frank aplastic anaemia, but haemolysis due to non-oxidative red cell destruction is also recognized. The exact mechanism for this is unknown. Penicillamine has also been described as causing a sideroblastic anaemia.
(iii) Blood loss due to multiple lacerations:
This has occurred, but is impossible to quantify.

Question 3: What further investigations are required to elucidate the cause of the anaemia?

Answer:
(a) Blood film with reticulocyte count – the red cells are normochromic and normocytic with a reticulocyte count of 2%.
(b) Haptoglobins – normal.
(c) Coombs' test – negative.
(d) Urobilinogen – positive.
(e) Liver function tests
    Bilirubin   35μmol/l
    Alkaline phosphatase   120u/l
    Total protein 66g/l
    Albumin   45g/l
    Globulin   21g/l
    Aspartate aminotransferase   30u/l
    Alanine aminotransferase   35u/l
(f) Serum B_{12} >2000ng/l
   Folate   >20μg/l
(g) Serum iron   8μmol/l (normal range 9–27μmol/l)
   Serum ferritin 1034μg/l (normal range female 12–150μg/l)
   Transferrin   1.8g/l (normal range 2.0–4.0g/l)

Upper GI endoscopy was planned but postponed on sight of the other investigation results.

Case 19

Question 4: Explain these multiple abnormalities.

Answer: The raised bilirubin and positive urobilinogen test are consistent with RBC breakdown secondary to the extensive bruising and these would be expected to return to the normal range rapidly. The increased ferritin is a manifestation of the anaemia of chronic disorder (rheumatoid arthritis) in which there is reticuloendothelial sequestration of iron, leading to an 'RE block' of iron delivery for RBC production. This is reflected by a normochromic, normocytic anaemia with raised serum ferritin and low serum iron and transferrin.

Question 5: What further test is now required?

Answer: Bone marrow examination. The results showed the following:
The marrow was hypercellular with dysplastic features which included 'megaloblastoid' erythropoiesis, nuclear irregularity and fragmentation and cytoplasmic vacuolation. There was also dysmegakaryopoiesis with large mononuclear forms and other nuclear aberrations. Occasional blast cells were seen and there were very occasional ringed sideroblasts on Prussian blue staining. This is the typical appearance of a myelodysplastic syndrome.

COMMENT

Myelodysplastic syndromes (MDS) are conditions of unknown cause in which there is progressive cytopenia, associated with a normocellular or hypercellular marrow and ineffectual haemopoeisis. It is usual for at least two of the cell lines to be involved out of the red cells or white cells and platelets. The definition exludes cytopenias due to aplasia of the marrow or to excessive peripheral destruction.

The majority of cases are labelled as primary MDS as no cause has been identified. They usually affect the elderly – median age 60–70 years. Some cases result from the treatment of lymphomas, multiple myeloma and related haematological malignancies with radiotherapy and chemotherapy (particularly alkylating agents). In this secondary type there is a significant incidence of subsequent development of acute myeloblastic leukaemia. Persons affected are usually younger and have been treated for prolonged periods. A new classification of primary MDS is shown in Table 1.

The myelodysplastic syndromes (MDS) are insidious, irreversible, progressive clonal disorders affecting all haemopoietic cell lines. Affected stem cells produce differentiated descendants that mature, but yield cells that are functionally and structurally defective. The cloned cells gradually replace normal haemopoietic cells leading to progressive cytopenias, ineffective erythropoiesis and, paradoxically, a hypercellular marrow pattern.

The clinical presentations are therefore usually anaemia, infections and fever or bleeding.

This patient presented with anaemia and excessive bleeding and bruising following trauma. At the initial evaluation she had several possible causes of anaemia including blood loss from chronic gastric ulcer or resulting from NSAID therapy, long standing rheumatoid arthritis and marrow suppression resulting from penicillamine therapy. Trauma induced excessive bleeding in a patient who was already thrombocytopenic. The diagnosis was confirmed as a refractory anaemia (RAB type) by the marrow findings (see Table 1). The haemoglobin had fallen after admission as she had haemodiluted following her blood loss and as her marrow function was so abnormal.

Table 1 Myelodysplastic syndromes

This new classification has been devised by a French, American and British co-operative group (FAB). It is based on findings in the peripheral blood and the bone marrow.

Classification	% Marrow blasts	% Peripheral blood blasts	Ringed sideroblasts
Refractory anaemia (RA)	<5	<1	0
Refractory anaemia with ringed sideroblasts (RAB)	<5	<1	+
Refractory anaemia with excess blasts (RAEB)	5–20	<5	+/–
RAEB in transition (RAEB-t)	20–30	>5	+/–
Chronic myelomonocytic leukaemia	<20	<5	+/–

The prognosis in such patients is reflected by the patient's age (it is worse in patients over 60 years), the severity of the marrow dysplasia, the selectivity and degree of cytopenia, the FAB classification from the bone marrow and any chromosomal abnormalities.

The most common causes of death in MDS relate to the presence of bleeding (from thrombocytopenia) or infection from neutropenia.

Anabolic steroids and glucocorticoids have been shown to have no place in management. Clinical trials are continuing with agents which promote cell differentiation, e.g. cis-retinoic acid, 1,25 dihydroxy vitamin D_3 and cytosine arabinoside. Prophylaxis against bacterial and fungal infections may also be needed.

CASE 20:
An Elderly Man with Breathlessness and Syncope

A previously active 82-year-old man was sent to the Emergency Department at 3 a.m. having woken up with acute breathlessness so severe that he had to get out of bed and sit on a chair at the open window. There had been similar, less severe, episodes on the three previous nights. He gave a 6 month history of tirednesss, breathlessness on exertion and orthopnoea. Recently he had noticed dizziness on occasions especially while walking upstairs to his bedroom. There was no past history of ischaemic heart disease or of any other relevant illness.

On examination he was breathless at rest with tachypnoea (35/min) and slight central cyanosis, but there was no peripheral oedema. The pulse rate was 110/min and regular; the jugular veins were not elevated; the heart sounds were probably normal but somewhat obscured by his dyspnoea. No murmurs were audible. There were bilateral crepitations over the lower half of both lung fields.

Question 1: What is the provisional clinical diagnosis?

Answer: Acute paroxysmal nocturnal dyspnoea – cause unknown at this stage.

Question 2: Fig. 1 is the chest X-ray taken on admission. What does it show?

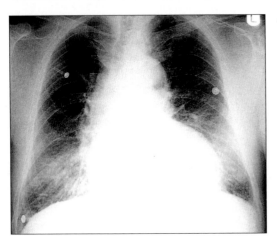

◀ **1** Chest X-ray (AP) on admission.

Answer: Gross cardiomegaly. Bilateral symmetrical increase in bronchovascular markings, especially in the lower zones. Bilateral Kerley B lines consistent with pulmonary oedema.

He was treated with 28% oxygen via a face mask, and intravenous frusemide. His clinical condition improved rapidly following diuresis so that later in the morning he was no longer breathless at rest.

Question 3: Fig. 2 is the ECG taken that morning. What does it show?

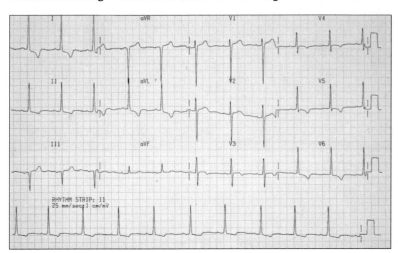

▲ 2 ECG recorded 6 hours after admission.

Answer: The ECG shows high voltages in the QRS complexes and down-sloping ST depression with T wave inversion in the left ventricular leads. This is the pattern of left ventricular hypertrophy and strain.

Question 4: Some aspects of the history and of these initial investigations raise the possibility of a specific cause for his acute pulmonary oedema. What are these aspects; what condition should be suspected; and which further investigation should he have?

Answer: The history of syncope on exertion, the chest X-ray and the ECG suggesting left ventricular hypertrophy all raise the possibility of aortic stenosis. He should have echocardiography including Doppler flow studies.

Question 5: Figs 3–6 illustrate the echo/Doppler appearances. What do they show?

Case 20

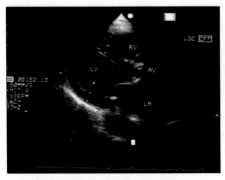

▲ **3** Echocardiogram (parasternal long axis view). RV = right ventricle; LV = left ventricle; AV = letters positioned to the right of the aortic valve; LA = left atrium.

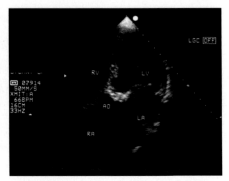

▲ **4** Echocardiogram (apical 4 chamber view). RV = right ventricle; LV = left ventricle; AO = aorta; RA = right atrium; LA = left atrium.

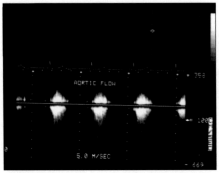

▲ **5** Doppler flow study of aortic valve.

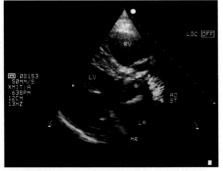

▲ **6** Colour flow Doppler echocardiogram (parasternal long axis view). RV = right ventricle; LV = left ventricle; AO = aorta; LA = left atrium.

Answer: The echo pictures (**Figs 3 & 4**) confirm the presence of left ventricular hypertrophy. The aortic valve is heavily calcified. The Doppler study (**Fig. 5**) shows a mosaic pattern at the aortic valve suggesting the valve is narrowed. The velocity of blood flow across the valve is 5 metres per second which gives an estimated valve gradient of 100mmHg. The appearances are very suggestive of significant aortic stenosis. The typical jet flow through the stenotic aortic valve is seen in **Fig. 6** (AO ST). **Fig. 6** also shows a minor degree of mitral regurgitation (MR).

COMMENT

The absence of a cardiac murmur does not exclude aortic stenosis as a possible diagnosis, especially if tachycardia or loud breath sounds are present, as they can obscure the murmur. Sometimes, even with a normal heart rate and quiet breathing, there is simply no murmur audible – the term 'occult aortic stenosis' is used to describe the condition. It is very important not to miss this diagnosis, which should always be borne in mind when a patient presents with either acute or chronic heart failure with no other obvious cause. In this patient's case the absence of ischaemic heart disease in the past and a history of dizziness on exertion should alert one to the possibility of aortic stenosis, which is supported by the fact that the ECG and CXR both show left ventricular enlargement.

The treatment of heart failure due to aortic stenosis is different from the treatment for that due primarily to myocardial failure. Agents which lower afterload, such as angiotensin converting enzyme inhibitors and nitrates, may increase the gradient across the valve and are relatively contraindicated. If aortic stenosis is sufficiently severe to cause cardiac failure urgent aortic valve replacement should be considered, as the prognosis with medical therapy alone is very poor.

The fact that this patient is 82 is obviously a factor in considering his suitability for surgery. However, as he was otherwise fit, age itself did not preclude him from surgery; indeed there is increasing evidence that octogenarians often do very well following aortic valve surgery.

CASE 21:
Weight Loss and Neglect in an Old Lady

A 76-year-old very neglected female was admitted via her family doctor as a case of acute onset pneumonia. However, on closer questioning it was apparent that she had not been really well for some time. Some 3 years earlier she had been widowed and as a result had become depressed and reclusive, shunning the company of neighbours and friends. Since then she had neglected her garden, house and herself and had resisted attempts by her doctor to involve social services. Her behaviour had also been rather unusual and this had further isolated her socially.

On admission she gave a history of pleuritic right sided chest pain which had been present for a couple of weeks and had become intolerable over the last few days. She had also had a dry, non-productive cough for some considerable time but had not coughed up any blood. She had suffered from chronic obstructive pulmonary disease (COPD) for some years and often had a cough with yellow–green sputum, especially in the winter. She had smoked up to 30 cigarettes per day 'all her life'. Recently she had become more short of breath, even on doing the household chores, and now rarely left the house. She said that she was always profoundly tired and often slept for long periods in the day in her chair. She rarely watched television and if she did she never remained awake long enough to see the end of the films. She complained bitterly of the cold and blamed this on her financial status which allowed her to heat only one room. She thought she had lost weight over the previous few months, and she put this down to her lack of appetite, which was also compounded by her immobility and inability to get out shopping.

Examination showed a thin, pallid old lady who had evidence of recent weight loss, looked ill, was clearly anaemic and had some obvious facial features of hypothyroidism – coarse hair, cold dry skin, myoedema and hoarseness of voice. She was running a low grade pyrexia of 38.4°C. There was an obvious herpes simplex lesion on her lip which she said had been present for at least a week (Fig. 1) and similar lesions were present on her tongue. There was early finger clubbing but no lymphadenopathy, cyanosis or peripheral oedema.

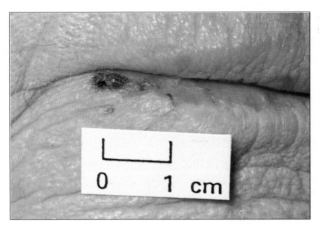

◀ **1** A 'cold sore' (herpes simplex) on the patient's lip.

The pulse rate was 60/min, the blood pressure was 110/55mmHg, the jugular venous pressure was not raised and examination of the heart was normal. Examination of the chest showed that the trachea was central, there were diminished movements on the right side with dullness to percussion over the right base (over which there was bronchial breathing), decreased air entry and coarse 'sticky' crepitations in the right mid and lower zones. No abdominal masses could be felt.

Question 1: What are the provisional diagnoses?

Answer: (a) Acute onset pneumonia of unknown cause, on the background of smoking and COPD. The possibility of lung cancer must be borne in mind.
(b) Hypothyroidism.
(c) Malnutrition.

The following initial screening investigations were carried out.

Haematology	Haemoglobin	11.5g/dl
	Haematocrit	0.352
	MCV	86.3fl
	MCH	28.9pg
	MCHC	33.5g/dl
	WBC	$37 \times 10^9/l$
	Platelets	$105 \times 10^9/l$
	ESR	135mm in 1st hour

Blood film: the red cells are normochromic, normocytic. There is neutrophilia with dysplastic, hypogranular neutrophils and a minor population of abnormal monocytes

Biochemistry

Sodium	122mmol/l	Bilirubin	8µmol/l
Potassium	3.5mmol/l	Total protein	79g/l
Chloride	85mmol/l	Albumin	47g/l
Bicarbonate	23mmol/l	Globulins	32g/l
Glucose (Random)	5.8mmol/l	Alkaline phosphatase	71u/l
		T4	40nmol/l
		TSH	17.3mU/l

ECG See Fig. 2
X-ray chest See Fig. 3

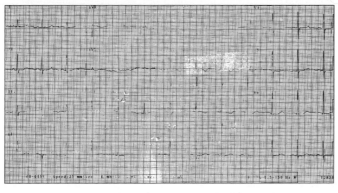

◀ **2** The ECG on admission.

Case 21

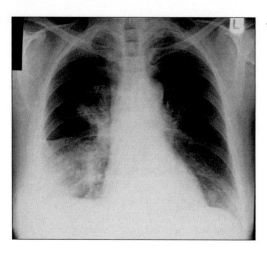

◀ **3** The chest X-ray on admission.

Question 2: Comment on these initial results.

Answer: The patient has normochromic, normocytic anaemia with a high white cell count that includes dysplastic cells, which suggest a myelodysplastic syndrome with thrombocytopenia. The ESR is extremely high and points to significant disease being present. Biochemical results show hyponatraemia, with low level of chloride, bicarbonate, urea and creatinine. The low level of T4 and the high TSH levels are diagnostic of hypothyroidism and confirm the clinical suspicion. The ECG shows minor ischaemia in the anterio-septal leads, but not the low voltage features sometimes seen in hypothyroidism.

The chest X-ray shows some enlargement of the right hilum and patchy consolidation of the right lower zone.

Question 3: What treatment should be instigated while the investigations continue?

Answer: (1) A broad spectrum intravenous antibiotic should be commenced (e.g. amoxycillin).

(2) The total fluid intake should be restricted to about 500ml per day (i.e. fluid intake to be less than urine output). The electrolyte profile should be carefully monitored.

(3) Treatment for the hypothyroidism may be cautiously started with thyroxine 50μg/day.

Despite antibiotic therapy she continued to have a swinging fever and her clinical condition did not improve. The white cell count rose to 72 × 10⁹/l with the same appearances as before on the blood film. Blood cultures and sputum sent at the time of admission grew no pathogens. Bronchoscopy was therefore undertaken and this confirmed the presence of pus in the bronchi in the right middle and lower lobes. A direct smear of this is shown in Fig. 4.

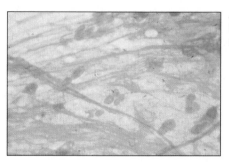

◀ **4** A smear of pus obtained from the right lower lobe bronchus, stained by a special method.

Question 4: What stain has been used and what is the cause of the pneumonia?

Answer: This is a Ziehl–Neelsen stain showing acid and alcohol-fast bacilli, confirming the presence of tuberculosis. Culture was also undertaken on Lowenstein–Jensen medium to determine the characteristics and sensitivity of the infecting organism.

Question 5: What first- and second-line drugs should be considered for the treatment of tuberculosis in this patient?

Answer: Anti-tuberculosis drugs:

First line	Second line
Rifampicin	Ethionamide
Isoniazid	Prothionamide
Ethambutol	Cycloserine
Pyrazinamide	Kanamycin
Streptomycin	Capreomycin
Thiacetazone	Viomycin
p-amino salicylic acid (PAS)	

In the event, she was started on rifampicin 600mg per day, isoniazid 300mg/day, and ethambutol 25mg/kg/day.

In a short time her hyponatraemia resolved and the total white cell count fell to $20 \times 10^9/l$. However she suddenly developed a diffuse, non-itchy, erythematous rash, which included larger lesions with central blistering. This was present over the hands, feet and trunk. This is shown in Fig. 5.

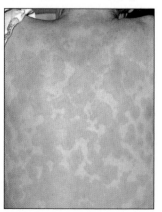

◀ **5** The skin rash which appeared after the start of therapy. Similar lesions were present on the patient's hands and feet.

Case 21

Question 6: What is the skin lesion? What are the common causes of this?

Answer: This is erythema multiforme. The typical 'target' lesions are well seen, and each characteristically blisters at the centre. In up to half the patients the cause is unknown. It may result from a range of virus infections (including herpes simplex, which she had), from infections with other organisms including streptococci and mycoplasma, and as a reaction to drug therapy, especially with sulphonamides. The prime suspect in this case was rifampicin which was stopped and replaced with streptomycin. The rash faded rapidly over the next few days.

Question 7: Does her white cell count merit further investigation?

Answer: Yes. A 'baseline' total white cell count of $20 \times 10^9/l$ is very high. The blood film points to a possible myelodysplastic disorder, so bone marrow aspiration is indicated.

COMMENT

Tuberculosis is a disease of great antiquity and is found worldwide. It is commonly associated with social deprivation, poor unhygienic housing, overcrowding and poor nutrition. Major efforts in the public health field over the past 100 years plus a public policy for immunization, screening and treatment led to a highly significant decline in prevalence in developed countries so that it became a rarity, being found mainly in new immigrants (usually from Asia or Africa), and as a reactivation of latent disease in the elderly, in alcoholics, in diabetics and in those treated with steroids or other immunosuppressive agents. In the last 10 years there has been an increasing incidence in patients who are immunocompromised by HIV infection. Worldwide there has been a dramatic reversal of the decline of this disease, due not only to the advent of HIV infection but also to wars, social disturbance and the resurgence of poverty due to political chaos.

The infecting organism is *Mycobacterium tuberculosis*, which is spread mainly by droplets which, when inhaled into the lungs or swallowed produce a characteristic granulomatous lesion with central caseation and multinucleated giant cells (Langhans' cells). The lung, alimentary tract and related lymph nodes are commonly involved in the primary process, which is most commonly seen in the young. The primary focus usually heals, but occasionally infection may spread by the blood to produce disseminated disease (miliary tuberculosis). The healed primary lesion encapsulates organisms which remain viable for many years – probably for the lifetime of the host. Within a few weeks of the primary infection, cell mediated immunity can be demonstrated, as shown by the development of a positive Mantoux test (the skin reaction to injected protein from the organism-purified protein derivative, P.P.D.).

In the elderly it is usually reactivation of these lesions that produces disease rather than reinfection from a new source. Reactivation may be associated with an intercurrent disease in which the patient's immunity declines. This old lady's presentation was typical, with a short history of an unproductive cough, breathlessness on exertion and later at rest, fever at night and progressive weight loss. She also had a history of heavy smoking and chronic obstructive pulmonary disease. She had been widowed for 3 years and had become reclusive and neglected. This may have been partly due to the onset of hypothyroidism, which may alter behaviour patterns. In addition, the bone marrow examination showed her to have chronic myelomonocytic leukaemia, which may also have caused perturbation of her background immunity and been partly responsible for reactivation of the lesions.

Examination on admission showed the presence of a herpes simplex lesion on her lip. This is often associated with acute onset pneumonia but may also point to declining immunity.

Her failure to respond to initial therapy for her pneumonia is not surprising. Sputum and blood cultures were unhelpful and direct smears of sputum stained by the Ziehl–Neelsen method were negative. The suggestive history with weight loss and night sweats plus failure to respond to an intravenous broad spectrum antibiotic, plus the very high ESR, encouraged the search for another cause of the pneumonia. The patient was bronchoscoped, and the sputum aspirated from the right lower lobe bronchus was found to contain alcohol and acid fast bacilli (Fig. 4).

Until recently, chronic myelomonocytic leukaemia (CMML) was classified with myelodysplastic syndromes (see p. 114) because the marrow appearances are similar to those in refractory anaemia with an excess of blasts (RAEB) but with the additional prominence of promonocytes. The incidence of CMML within MDS is between 5 and 20%. The peripheral blood appearances, as in this patient, are characterized by neutrophilia and monocytosis ($>1 \times 10^9$/l) and there is usually thrombocytopenia of sufficient degree to cause bleeding. CMML is a disease usually affecting the elderly which runs a very chronic course, usually over a few years. There may be evolution to acute myeloid leukaemia (up to 25% of patients). In up to 20% of cases there may be splenomegaly but this was not a feature in this patient.

Treatment for her tuberculosis was started with a triple therapy regimen of rifampicin, isoniazid and ethambutol. Rifampicin is the drug of choice in this combination as it is bactericidal. It is well tolerated, is well absorbed from the alimentary tract, rapidly reaches an effective serum level and diffuses into most tissues. The metabolic product is desacetyl rifampicin which gives a pink colour to the body secretions (urine, faeces, tears etc). It is excreted mainly in the bile, with 10% in urine. Because it is a hepatic enzyme inducer care should be taken when other drugs are given concomitantly. The daily dose for a 70kg adult is 600mg. Rifampicin is generally an extremely safe and effective drug with only occasional serious side effects, usually manifested in the skin, gut, liver and bone marrow. In this patient a severe rash developed 2 weeks after starting combination therapy. The rash was thought to be erythema multiforme because the lesions were typically target shaped with central blistering and because of the classical distribution involving hands, feet and trunk. The rash rapidly settled when rifampicin was withdrawn.

Isoniazid is a proven, effective, and relatively safe drug which can be used in combination with rifampicin. The daily dose is 300mg. It is bactericidal, has excellent alimentary absorption and a rapidly effective therapeutic level. It also diffuses easily into all tissues. There is an excellent safety profile, but at high doses peripheral neuropathy, optic neuritis, and encephalopathy may be produced, probably as a result of pyridoxine deficiency in those people who are slow acetylators of the drug and in whom the half-life is significantly prolonged. Pyridoxine 10mg/day should be given routinely to all patients treated with isoniazid.

Ethambutol is a bacteriostatic drug and is used in combination with other bactericidal drugs to prevent the emergence of resistant strains. It is readily absorbed after oral dosage. Caution must be used in the presence of renal failure as this results in high serum levels and may result in retro-bulbar neuritis. The usual dose is 25mg/kg/day.

Following the onset of the skin rash and withdrawal of rifampicin the patient was started on streptomycin, an aminoglycoside antibiotic which is bactericidal. The dose was 150mg/day, and this reduced dosage was chosen because of the patient's age.

Index

Index